EVELIN OIMANDI

Out of My Mind: Navigating Brain Health

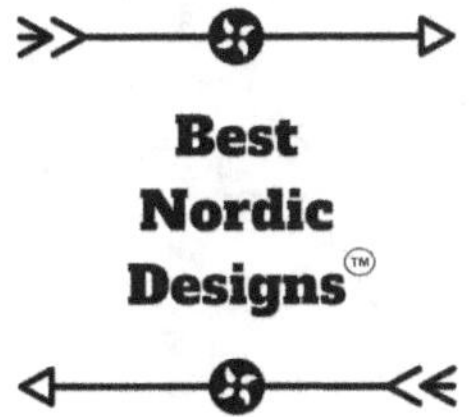

Contents

Foreword

Introduction

Brain health is something that affects all of us, yet it's a topic that we often avoid discussing. We often think of brain health as something that only concerns individuals who have suffered from brain injuries, such as strokes or concussions. However, the truth is that brain health is something that we should all prioritize, regardless of our age or current health status. In "Out of My Mind: Navigating Brain Health," we'll explore the importance of brain health, ways to maintain a healthy brain, and how to cope with the challenges of brain-related conditions.

Chapter 1: The Basics of Brain Health

In this chapter, we'll cover the basics of brain health. We'll explore what the brain does, how it works, and why it's important to keep it healthy. We'll also delve into common brain-related conditions, such as Alzheimer's disease, Parkinson's disease, and depression, and discuss the impact they have on the brain and overall health.

Chapter 2: Lifestyle Choices and Brain Health

In this chapter, we'll focus on how lifestyle choices impact brain health. We'll explore the importance of regular exercise, a healthy diet, and quality sleep in maintaining a healthy brain. We'll also discuss the impact of stress, drug and alcohol use, and other factors that can have negative effects on brain health.

Chapter 3: Coping with Brain-Related Conditions

In this chapter, we'll explore the challenges of coping with brain-related conditions. We'll discuss the impact of these conditions on mental health, and provide coping strategies for individuals and their loved ones. We'll also discuss the importance of seeking professional help and support when dealing with brain-related conditions.

Chapter 4: Brain Health and Aging

In this chapter, we'll explore the relationship between brain health and aging. We'll discuss common age-related conditions, such as dementia, and provide tips for maintaining a healthy brain as we age. We'll also discuss the importance of staying mentally active and socially engaged as we grow older.

Chapter 5: The Future of Brain Health

In this final chapter, we'll explore the future of brain health. We'll discuss new technologies and treatments that are being developed to improve brain health and treat brain-related conditions. We'll also discuss the importance of ongoing research and education in promoting brain health.

Conclusion

In "Out of My Mind: Navigating Brain Health," we've explored the importance of brain health, ways to maintain a healthy brain, and how to cope with brain-related conditions. By prioritizing brain health and making positive lifestyle choices, we can all improve our overall health and well-being.

1

Chapter 1: The Basics of Brain Health

"Take care of your brain, and your brain will take care of you." - Amen Clinics

* * *

The brain is a complex and remarkable organ that controls our thoughts, feelings, and behaviors. It is the center of our nervous system, and its health is critical to our overall well-being. In this chapter, we will explore the basics of brain health, including what it is, why it matters, and how we can maintain it.[1]

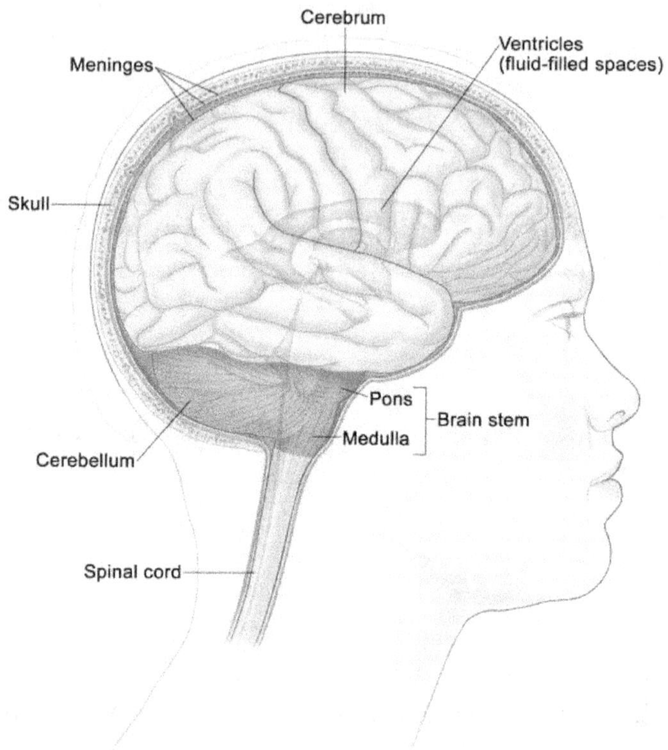

Drawing of brain anatomy showing the brain stem, pons, medulla, spinal cord, cerebellum, cerebrum, meninges, ventricles (fluid-filled spaces), and skull.[2]

The brain is an organ responsible for a wide range of cognitive and physiological functions. It is composed of several structures that work in conjunction to ensure optimal performance.

The brain can be divided into several main regions, including the cerebrum, cerebellum, and brain stem. The cerebrum is the largest and most complex part of the brain and is responsible for conscious thought, learning, and memory. It is further divided into two hemispheres, each of which is responsible for specific functions. The left hemisphere is responsible for language, logical thinking, and analytical skills, while the right hemisphere is associated with creativity, spatial awareness, and emotional processing.[3]

The cerebellum, located at the base of the brain, is responsible for balance, posture, and coordination. The brain stem, which connects the brain to the spinal cord, is responsible for regulating vital functions such as breathing, heart rate, and blood pressure.[4]

Within each of these regions, there are numerous structures that work together to ensure optimal function. For example, the cerebrum contains several lobes, each of which is associated with specific functions. The frontal lobe is responsible for decision-making, planning, and problem-solving, while the temporal lobe is associated with memory and hearing.

Additionally, the brain is composed of several types of cells, including neurons and glial cells. Neurons are responsible for transmitting electrical signals throughout the brain, while glial cells provide support and protection to neurons.[5]

What is Brain Health?

Brain health refers to the overall state of our brain, including its structure, function, and performance. It encompasses everything from the physical health of the brain, such as the integrity of its neurons and synapses, to the mental health of the individual, such as their emotional stability and cognitive function.

Why Does Brain Health Matter?

Our brain health is essential because it affects every aspect of our lives, including our ability to think, learn, remember, and communicate. It also plays a significant role in our emotional well-being, impacting our moods, behaviors, and relationships. Additionally, brain health is crucial in preventing and managing neurological disorders such as Alzheimer's disease, Parkinson's disease, and epilepsy.[6]

Numerous studies have demonstrated the importance of brain health. For example, research has shown that poor brain health is a major risk factor for cognitive decline and dementia in older adults[7]. Additionally, studies have found that individuals with mental health disorders, such as depression and anxiety, have altered brain function and structure[8]. Moreover, poor brain health can also have physical consequences, such as an increased risk of stroke and cardiovascular disease[9].

Factors that can influence brain health include genetics, lifestyle factors, and environmental factors. For example, genetics play a significant role in determining an individual's risk of developing certain neurological conditions, such as Alzheimer's disease[10]. Lifestyle factors, such as diet, exercise, and sleep, can also impact brain health. For instance, studies have found that exercise can improve cognitive function and reduce the risk of cognitive decline[11]. Environmental factors, such as exposure to toxins and pollutants, can also impact brain health. For example, studies have found that exposure to air pollution is associated with cognitive decline and dementia[12].

In summary, brain health is a critical aspect of overall health and well being. Poor brain health can have serious consequences, such as cognitive decline, mental health disorders, and physical ailments. Factors that influence brain health include genetics, lifestyle factors, and environmental factors. However, individuals can take steps to maintain and improve brain health through lifestyle changes and engaging in activities that challenge the brain.

How Can We Maintain Brain Health?

Maintaining brain health involves a variety of strategies, including physical activity, healthy eating, and cognitive stimulation. Let's explore each of these strategies in more detail.

Physical Activity

Physical activity is an essential component of brain health. It has been shown to improve cognitive function, increase blood flow to the brain, and promote the growth of new neurons. Exercise also helps to reduce the risk of developing neurological disorders such as dementia and Alzheimer's disease.[13]

Physical activity has long been recognized as a crucial component of a healthy lifestyle. Regular exercise has been associated with a reduced risk of chronic diseases, improved cardiovascular health, and weight management. However, emerging evidence also suggests that physical activity is vital for brain health. Physical activity has been linked to improved cognitive function, reduced risk of neurodegenerative diseases, and enhanced brain plasticity.[14]

The Importance of Physical Activity for Brain Health

Physical activity has been found to have several beneficial effects on the brain. Exercise has been shown to enhance cognitive function, improve memory and learning, and increase brain plasticity. Regular exercise can also reduce the risk of neurodegenerative diseases such as Alzheimer's disease and Parkinson's disease.

One study found that regular physical activity was associated with a reduced risk of cognitive decline in older adults. The study followed a group of older adults for six years and found that those who engaged in regular physical activity had better cognitive function than those who were sedentary.[15]

Another study found that exercise can increase brain plasticity. Brain plasticity refers to the brain's ability to change and adapt in response to new experiences. Exercise has been shown to increase the production of growth factors that promote the growth of new neurons and synapses, which are the connections between neurons.[16]

Physical activity has also been linked to a reduced risk of neurodegenerative diseases. One study found that regular exercise was associated with a reduced risk of Alzheimer's disease. The study followed a group of older adults for five years and found that those who engaged in regular physical activity had a lower risk of developing Alzheimer's disease than those who were sedentary.[17]

Healthy Eating

A healthy diet is critical to brain health. Nutrients such as omega-3 fatty acids, antioxidants, and B vitamins have been shown to improve cognitive function and protect against neurological damage. Additionally, reducing the intake of processed foods and added sugars has been linked to a reduced risk of cognitive decline.[18]

Healthy eating is an essential component of brain health, as the brain is a metabolically active organ that requires a constant supply of nutrients to function properly. The food we eat provides the building blocks for neurotransmitters, which are essential for communication between brain cells. Additionally, research has shown that specific nutrients and dietary patterns can directly influence brain health and cognition[19].

One critical nutrient for brain health is omega-3 fatty acids, which are found in fatty fish, nuts, and seeds. Omega-3s are crucial for the development and maintenance of brain cells, as well as for the regulation of inflammation in the brain. A systematic review of randomized controlled trials found that omega-3 supplementation improved cognitive function in healthy adults and those with mild cognitive impairment[20].

Another essential nutrient for brain health is choline, which is found in foods such as eggs, liver, and soybeans. Choline is a precursor for acetylcholine, a neurotransmitter that plays a crucial role in learning and memory. A study of healthy adults found that higher dietary choline intake was associated with better cognitive performance.[21]

Furthermore, research suggests that specific dietary patterns, such as the Mediterranean diet, may be protective against cognitive decline and dementia. The Mediterranean diet is rich in fruits, vegetables, whole grains, and healthy fats, such as olive oil and nuts. A meta-analysis of observational studies found that adherence to the Mediterranean diet was associated with a lower risk of cognitive decline and Alzheimer's disease.[22]

In contrast, a Western-style diet, which is high in processed and fried foods, refined grains, and sugar, has been linked to poorer cognitive function and an increased risk of dementia. A longitudinal study of older adults found that higher adherence to a Western-style diet was associated with a greater decline in cognitive function over a four-year period.[23]

In summary, healthy eating is essential for brain health, as specific nutrients and dietary patterns can directly influence brain function and cognition. Adequate intake of omega-3 fatty acids and choline, as well as adherence to a healthy dietary pattern such as the Mediterranean diet, may help to protect against cognitive decline and dementia.

Cognitive Stimulation

Cognitive stimulation refers to activities that challenge the brain, such as reading, learning a new skill, or playing a musical instrument. These activities have been shown to improve cognitive function and protect against neurological decline. Additionally, social engagement and maintaining strong relationships have been linked to better cognitive function and a reduced risk of developing neurological disorders.[24]

One reason why cognitive stimulation is essential for brain health is that it can help to maintain and improve cognitive function. A study by Wilson et al.[25] found that older adults who engaged in more cognitive activities had a lower risk of developing Alzheimer's disease and other forms of dementia. Similarly, a study by Valenzuela and Sachdev[26] found that cognitive training can improve cognitive function in older adults, particularly in areas such as memory and executive function.

Cognitive stimulation is also essential for preventing cognitive decline. A longitudinal study by Salthouse et al.[27] found that engaging in cognitively stimulating activities was associated with slower rates of cognitive decline in older adults. Similarly, a systematic review by Hill et al.[28] found that cognitive training can improve cognitive function and reduce the risk of cognitive decline in older adults.

In addition to maintaining and improving cognitive function, cognitive stimulation can also improve brain function in older adults. A study by Lövdén et al.[29] found that cognitive training can improve brain structure and function in older adults, particularly in areas such as the prefrontal cortex and hippocampus. Similarly, a study by Kelly et al.[30] found that cognitive training can improve white matter integrity in older adults, which is important for communication between different parts of the brain.

Overall, the evidence suggests that cognitive stimulation is an essential component of brain health. Engaging in activities that challenge and stimulate the brain can help to maintain cognitive function, prevent cognitive decline, and even improve brain function in older adults. As such, cognitive stimulation should be promoted as a key strategy for promoting brain health and preventing cognitive decline in older adults.

Conclusion

Maintaining brain health is critical to our overall well-being.

Physical activity, healthy eating, and cognitive stimulation are all essential components of brain health. By taking care of our brain, we can improve our cognitive function, protect against neurological disorders, and enhance our overall quality of life.

2

Chapter 2: Lifestyle Choices and Brain Health

"As I see it, every day you do one of two things: build health or produce disease in yourself." - Adelle Davis

* * *

Our brain is an incredible organ, responsible for almost everything we do, think, and feel. It requires a lot of energy to function properly, and our lifestyle choices can significantly impact its health and performance. In this chapter, we will explore how certain lifestyle choices, including diet, exercise, sleep, and stress management, can affect brain health.

Diet

The food we eat provides the fuel and building blocks for our body and brain. The brain is a metabolically active organ that requires a constant supply of energy to function correctly. The food we consume plays a vital role in maintaining brain health and function throughout our lifespan. In this chapter, we will discuss the impact of diet on brain health and cognition.

Mediterranean Diet and Brain Health

Several studies have shown that a healthy diet can reduce the risk of cognitive decline and dementia. The Mediterranean diet, which is rich in fruits, vegetables, whole grains, fish, and olive oil, has been associated with better cognitive function and lower risk of Alzheimer's disease. In a study by Scarmeas et al.[31], adherence to the Mediterranean diet was associated with a 28% reduction in the risk of developing Alzheimer's disease. Similarly, a study by Tangney et al.[32] found that adherence to the Mediterranean diet was associated with slower cognitive decline in older adults.

The Mediterranean diet is rich in antioxidants and anti-inflammatory compounds, which may protect against oxidative stress and inflammation in the brain. It is also high in omega-3 fatty acids, which are essential for brain health and function. Omega-3 fatty acids have been shown to improve cognitive function and reduce the risk of cognitive decline and dementia[33].

On the other hand, a diet high in saturated and trans fats, sugar, and processed foods has been linked to cognitive impairment and an increased risk of dementia. One study found that a diet high in saturated fats and sugar was associated with worse memory and smaller brain volume[34].

Sugar and Cognitive Function

Sugar is a major component of the Western diet and is associated with several health problems, including obesity, type 2 diabetes, and cardiovascular disease. It has also been linked to cognitive impairment and dementia. A study by Kerti et al.[35] found that a high sugar intake was associated with worse cognitive function and a smaller hippocampal volume in older adults. The hippocampus is a brain region that plays a critical role in learning and memory.

Sugar consumption has also been linked to inflammation in the brain, which can contribute to the development of cognitive decline and dementia. A study by Liu et al.[36] found that a high sugar diet increased inflammatory markers in the brain and impaired cognitive function in mice.

Conclusion

In conclusion, diet plays a crucial role in brain health and cognitive function. The Mediterranean diet, which is rich in fruits, vegetables, whole grains, fish, and olive oil, has been associated with better cognitive function and lower risk of Alzheimer's disease. On the other hand, a diet high in saturated and trans fats, sugar, and processed foods has been linked to cognitive impairment and an increased risk of dementia. Therefore, it is essential to adopt a healthy diet that is rich in nutrients and antioxidants to maintain brain health and function throughout our lifespan.

Physical Activity

Regular physical activity is essential for maintaining good physical and mental health, including brain health. Exercise has been shown to have a positive impact on cognitive function, brain plasticity, and the risk of dementia[37]. A meta-analysis of 11 randomized controlled trials found that exercise interventions improved cognitive function in healthy older adults, with the most significant benefits seen in executive function, processing speed, and working memory[38].

In addition to improving cognitive function, exercise has been linked to structural changes in the brain. A longitudinal study found that older adults who engaged in regular physical activity had larger brain volumes in regions associated with cognitive function compared to their sedentary peers[39]. Another study found that exercise increased gray matter volume in the pre-frontal cortex, a region critical for executive function[40].

Even light exercise, such as walking, can have benefits for brain health. A randomized controlled trial found that walking for 30 minutes a day, three times a week, improved cognitive function in older adults with mild cognitive impairment[41]. Other studies have also shown that regular walking is associated with reduced risk of cognitive decline and dementia [63].

In conclusion, regular physical activity, including light exercise such as walking, is crucial for maintaining good brain health. Exercise has been shown to improve cognitive function, promote brain plasticity, and reduce the risk of dementia. These findings highlight the importance of including physical activity as part of a comprehensive approach to brain health.

Sleep

Sleep is a fundamental aspect of brain health, with significant implications for cognitive function and overall well-being. Numerous studies have linked sleep deprivation to cognitive impairment, including difficulties with attention, working memory, and decision-making[42]. Additionally, sleep disruption has been shown to impair memory consolidation, a process critical for learning and retaining new information[43].

Furthermore, chronic sleep deprivation has been associated with an increased risk of developing dementia, a debilitating condition that affects cognitive and functional abilities[44] [45]. Studies have found that sleep problems, such as insomnia, are common in individuals with dementia and may contribute to the progression of the disease[46].

Research has also demonstrated that sleep deprivation can have structural effects on the brain. In a study of chronically sleep-deprived rats, it was found that the hippocampus, a region important for memory and learning, had a significant reduction in volume compared to control rats[47]. Similar results have been found in humans, with chronic sleep deprivation linked to decreased gray matter volume in the prefrontal cortex, a region important for executive function[48].

In conclusion, sleep is an essential component of brain health, with significant implications for cognitive function and overall well-being. Chronic sleep deprivation can lead to cognitive impairment, memory problems, and an increased risk of dementia. Furthermore, sleep deprivation can have structural effects on the brain, highlighting the importance of getting enough quality sleep for optimal brain function and health.

Stress Management

Chronic stress can have a negative impact on brain health. It has been linked to cognitive impairment, anxiety, and depression[49]. Chronic stress can also cause damage to the hippocampus, a region important for memory and learning[50].

Several stress management techniques, such as meditation, yoga, and mindfulness, have been shown to have positive effects on brain health. One study found that a mindfulness-based stress reduction program improved memory and cognitive function in older adults.[51][52]

Social Engagement

Social engagement is essential for brain health. Regular social interaction can reduce the risk of cognitive decline and Alzheimer's disease[53][54]. It also promotes emotional well-being, reducing the risk of depression and anxiety. Activities such as volunteering, joining clubs or groups, and spending time with friends and family can provide social engagement and promote brain health.[55]

Mental Stimulation

Mental stimulation is critical for brain health. Regularly challenging the brain through activities such as reading, puzzles, and learning new skills can promote cognitive function and reduce the risk of cognitive decline. Experts recommend engaging in mentally stimulating activities throughout life to maintain optimal brain health[56].

Conclusion

Our lifestyle choices can significantly impact brain health. A healthy diet, regular exercise, quality sleep, and effective stress management techniques can all promote brain health and reduce the risk of cognitive decline and dementia. It's never too late to make positive changes to improve brain health and function.

3

Chapter 3: Coping with Brain-Related Conditions

"One of the things I learned the hard way was that it doesn't pay to get discouraged. Keeping busy and making optimism a way of life can restore your faith in yourself." - Lucille Ball

* * *

When faced with a brain-related condition, coping can be challenging. A brain-related condition can affect different aspects of a person's life, including their physical, cognitive, and emotional well-being. Coping strategies can vary based on the specific condition and individual needs. In this chapter, we will explore some coping strategies for common brain-related conditions.

Traumatic Brain Injury

Traumatic brain injury (TBI) occurs when there is a sudden blow or jolt to the head that disrupts normal brain function. Symptoms can range from mild to severe and can include headache, nausea, confusion, loss of consciousness, and memory problems[57]. Coping with TBI can be challenging, but with the right strategies, it is possible to manage symptoms and improve quality of life. Here are some coping strategies that can help:

Follow a treatment plan

Following a treatment plan for TBI can help manage symptoms and promote recovery. Treatment plans can include medical treatment, rehabilitation, and therapy. Several studies have shown that following a treatment plan for TBI can significantly improve patient outcomes. In a randomized controlled trial, patients who received intensive rehabilitation had better cognitive function and quality of life than those who received standard care[58]. Similarly, a systematic review found that multidisciplinary rehabilitation programs can improve functional outcomes and reduce disability in TBI patients[59]. Thus, it is essential for individuals with TBI and their caregivers to work closely with healthcare professionals to develop and implement a comprehensive treatment plan that addresses their specific needs and goals.

Take care of yourself

Taking care of oneself is essential to manage TBI symptoms. Self-care can include getting enough rest, eating a balanced diet, and avoiding alcohol and drugs. Numerous studies have demonstrated the benefits of self-care in managing symptoms of TBI. For example, one study found that adequate sleep can improve cognitive function and reduce fatigue in TBI patients[60]. Additionally, a balanced diet rich in nutrients like omega-3 fatty acids has been shown to support brain health and promote recovery after TBI[61]. On the other hand, alcohol and drug use can exacerbate TBI symptoms and impair the brain's ability to heal[62]. Therefore, practicing self-care is an essential aspect of navigating brain health and promoting recovery after TBI.

Communicate with others

Communicating with others can help reduce feelings of isolation and provide emotional support. Communication can include talking to family and friends, participating in support groups, and seeking professional counseling. Research has shown that social support is essential for the recovery and management of TBI[63]. Communicating with others can help people with TBI reduce feelings of isolation and provide emotional support[64]. Family and friends play a critical role in the emotional well-being of individuals with TBI[65]. Participation in support groups and seeking professional counseling have also been found to be effective in managing the emotional and psychological impact of TBI[66]. Overall, communication can be an effective tool for individuals with TBI to navigate their brain health and improve their quality of life.

Stay positive

TBI recovery can be a long and challenging process, but staying positive can improve overall well-being. Positive thinking can include focusing on progress, setting achievable goals, and celebrating small victories.[67] Research has shown that positive thinking can have a significant impact on the recovery process after a TBI. According to a study by Schepers and colleagues[68], individuals with TBI who had a positive attitude towards their recovery had better functional outcomes than those with a negative attitude. Similarly, a review by Baguley and colleagues[69] found that positive thinking and optimism were associated with better physical and cognitive functioning after TBI. Therefore, while TBI recovery can be a long and challenging process, maintaining a positive mindset can be an important factor in achieving optimal well-being and outcomes. By focusing on progress, setting achievable goals, and celebrating small victories, individuals can cultivate a positive outlook that can help them navigate the challenges of TBI recovery with greater resilience and success.

Cognitive rehabilitation

One effective coping strategy for TBI is cognitive rehabilitation. Cognitive rehabilitation is a treatment approach that helps individuals with brain injuries improve cognitive abilities such as memory, attention, and problem-solving. Studies have shown that cognitive rehabilitation can improve cognitive function and overall quality of life for individuals with TBI[70]. Furthermore, research indicates that cognitive rehabilitation can result in significant changes in brain activity and neural connectivity, leading to improved outcomes for individuals with TBI[71] [72]. It is important to note that cognitive rehabilitation should be tailored to each individual's unique needs and goals, and may involve a combination of different strategies such as computer-based training, behavioral therapy, and medication management[73]. With proper assessment and implementation, cognitive rehabilitation can be a powerful tool for individuals with TBI to regain independence and improve their overall well-being.

Social support

Another effective coping strategy for TBI is social support. Social support can come from friends, family, or support groups. Having a support system can help individuals with TBI cope with the challenges of their condition and improve their mental health. A study by Al-Rashaida et al.[74] found that social support was positively associated with better quality of life for individuals with TBI. In addition, research has also shown that social support can lead to better cognitive functioning and improved physical health outcomes for individuals with TBI[75] [76]. Therefore, it is important for individuals with TBI to seek out and utilize social support as a key aspect of their coping and recovery process. As stated by one participant in a study on social support for individuals with TBI, "Having a support system is the key to not feeling alone in this journey"[77]. By building and maintaining a strong support system, individuals with TBI can navigate the challenges of their condition and improve their overall well-being.

Stroke

Stroke is a brain-related condition that occurs when the blood supply to the brain is interrupted, causing brain cells to die. Symptoms can include weakness on one side of the body, difficulty speaking, and vision problems. Coping with the aftermath of a stroke can be a challenging and daunting task. It can be difficult to adjust to the physical, emotional, and cognitive changes that can result from a stroke. However, there are strategies that can help stroke survivors and their caregivers navigate this journey more successfully. In this chapter, we will discuss some coping strategies for stroke, backed up by academic research.

Seek Social Support

Studies have shown that social support can help stroke survivors cope with the aftermath of a stroke. A systematic review of 15 studies found that social support was associated with better quality of life and psychological well-being among stroke survivors[78]. Social support can come in different forms, such as family, friends, support groups, and healthcare professionals. The importance of social support in stroke recovery cannot be overemphasized. According to a study conducted by Carod-Artal et al.[79], social support is an essential factor that can influence the outcome of stroke recovery. In their study, stroke survivors with higher levels of social support were found to have better functional outcomes, lower levels of depression and anxiety, and higher levels of satisfaction with life.

Furthermore, a study conducted by House et al.[80] found that social support can help buffer the negative effects of stress, which is a common experience for stroke survivors. The study suggested that social support can reduce the psychological distress associated with stress and help individuals cope with stress more effectively. This is particularly important for stroke survivors who may experience a range of stressors, such as physical limitations, communication difficulties, and changes in social roles and relationships.

One form of social support that has been found to be particularly beneficial for stroke survivors is support groups. Support groups provide a safe and supportive environment where stroke survivors can share their experiences, learn coping strategies, and receive emotional and practical support from others who have gone through similar experiences. A study conducted by Mihailidis et al.[81] found that stroke survivors who participated in a support group reported higher levels of social support, lower levels of depression and anxiety, and greater satisfaction with life compared to those who did not participate in a support group.

In addition to support groups, healthcare professionals also play a crucial role in providing social support to stroke survivors. Healthcare professionals can provide emotional support, education, and practical advice to stroke survivors and their families. A study conducted by Williams et al.[82] found that stroke survivors who received social support from healthcare professionals reported higher levels of satisfaction with their healthcare, higher levels of functional independence, and lower levels of depression compared to those who did not receive social support from healthcare professionals.

In conclusion, social support is a vital factor in stroke recovery and can have a significant impact on the quality of life and psychological well-being of stroke survivors. Social support can come in different forms, such as family, friends, support groups, and healthcare professionals, and should be an integral part of stroke rehabilitation programs. Stroke survivors and their families should be encouraged to seek out and utilize social support resources to facilitate their recovery and improve their overall well-being.

Participate in Rehabilitation Programs

Rehabilitation programs are designed to help stroke survivors regain their physical, emotional, and cognitive abilities. Stroke is a leading cause of long-term disability and affects approximately 15 million people worldwide each year[83]. Survivors of stroke often experience physical, emotional, and cognitive impairments that can significantly impact their quality of life. Fortunately, rehabilitation programs can help individuals with stroke regain their functional abilities and achieve their personal goals.

Physical Rehabilitation

Physical rehabilitation is a crucial component of stroke rehabilitation and involves various exercises and activities aimed at improving physical function. Physical rehabilitation programs can help stroke survivors regain strength, balance, and coordination, which are essential for performing everyday activities. Additionally, physical rehabilitation programs can reduce the risk of falls and other secondary complications.[84]

Studies have shown that physical rehabilitation can improve physical function and overall quality of life for individuals who have had a stroke[85]. A meta-analysis of 25 studies found that rehabilitation programs were associated with improved motor function, activities of daily living, and quality of life among stroke survivors[86]. The American Stroke Association recommends that stroke survivors receive at least three hours of physical rehabilitation per day, five days per week, for optimal recovery[87].

Emotional Rehabilitation

Stroke can also cause emotional impairments, including depression, anxiety, and a decreased sense of well-being. Emotional rehabilitation aims to help stroke survivors cope with the emotional impact of stroke and improve their overall mental health. Emotional rehabilitation programs can involve individual or group therapy, counseling, and support groups.

A systematic review of 15 studies found that emotional rehabilitation programs were associated with reduced depression and anxiety and improved quality of life among stroke survivors[88]. Moreover, emotional rehabilitation can help stroke survivors cope with the emotional challenges of living with a disability and improve their self-esteem and confidence.

Cognitive Rehabilitation

Cognitive impairments, such as memory loss, attention deficits, and language difficulties, are common among stroke survivors. Cognitive rehabilitation aims to improve cognitive function and help stroke survivors regain their cognitive abilities. Cognitive rehabilitation programs can involve various activities, such as memory exercises, problem-solving tasks, and language therapy.

A systematic review of 14 studies found that cognitive rehabilitation programs were associated with improved cognitive function and activities of daily living among stroke survivors[89].

Cognitive rehabilitation can also help stroke survivors adapt to their cognitive impairments and learn compensatory strategies to improve their functioning.

Tailored Rehabilitation Programs

It is essential to participate in a comprehensive rehabilitation program tailored to the individual's needs and goals. Rehabilitation programs should take into account the individual's age, sex, culture, and level of impairment to achieve optimal outcomes. Moreover, rehabilitation programs should involve a multidisciplinary team, including physicians, nurses, therapists, and social workers, to provide comprehensive care.

Rehabilitation programs are essential for stroke survivors to regain their physical, emotional, and cognitive abilities and improve their quality of life. Physical rehabilitation can improve physical function, emotional rehabilitation can improve mental health, and cognitive rehabilitation can improve cognitive function. Therefore, stroke survivors should participate in a comprehensive rehabilitation program tailored to their needs and goals to achieve optimal outcomes.

Practice Mindfulness-Based Interventions

Mindfulness-based interventions, which typically involve practices such as meditation, yoga, and tai chi, have gained popularity in recent years as a way to improve mental health and well-being. These practices involve training the mind to focus on the present moment, often through techniques such as deep breathing and body awareness. While mindfulness-based interventions have been studied extensively in various populations, including healthy individuals and those with mental health conditions, their potential benefits for stroke survivors are particularly noteworthy.

Stroke survivors often experience a range of physical and psychological challenges as a result of their condition. In addition to physical disabilities such as weakness and difficulty with mobility, stroke survivors may also experience cognitive impairment, depression, anxiety, and other mental health issues. Mindfulness-based interventions have the potential to address many of these challenges by improving emotional regulation, reducing stress and anxiety, and enhancing cognitive functioning.

A systematic review of 11 studies conducted by Lawrence et al.[90] examined the effectiveness of mindfulness-based interventions among stroke survivors. The review found that these interventions were associated with improved psychological well-being, including reduced symptoms of depression and anxiety, as well as improved quality of life. Additionally, mindfulness-based interventions were found to improve attention, cognitive flexibility, and working memory among stroke survivors[91].

Several individual studies have also explored the potential benefits of specific mindfulness-based interventions for stroke survivors. For example, a randomized controlled trial by Liu et al.[92] found that a mindfulness-based stress reduction program was associated with improved mental health outcomes and quality of life among stroke survivors. Similarly, a pilot study by Wang et al.[93] found that a tai chi program was associated with improved balance, mobility, and cognitive function among stroke survivors.

While the evidence supporting the potential benefits of mindfulness-based interventions for stroke survivors is still relatively limited, the available research suggests that these interventions may be a promising approach to improving mental health and cognitive functioning in this population. As with any intervention, it is important to work with a healthcare provider to determine whether mindfulness-based interventions are appropriate and safe for an individual stroke survivor. However, given the potential benefits, mindfulness based interventions may be a valuable tool in helping stroke survivors navigate the challenges of post-stroke recovery and improve their overall well-being.

Set realistic goals

Stroke can significantly impact an individual's life and cause physical, emotional, and cognitive changes. The process of recovery can be long and challenging, and it is essential to set realistic goals to regain a sense of control and purpose in life. In this chapter, we will explore the importance of goal-setting for stroke survivors and the benefits of involving the stroke survivor and their caregiver in the process. We will also discuss the characteristics of effective goals and provide tips for setting and achieving them.

Importance of Goal-Setting for Stroke Survivors

Goal-setting is a crucial aspect of stroke rehabilitation. It enables the stroke survivor to focus on their strengths, abilities, and interests, rather than their limitations. Setting realistic goals can improve the stroke survivor's motivation, self-confidence, and overall quality of life[94]. Goals also help the stroke survivor to track their progress and celebrate their achievements, no matter how small.

Involving the Stroke Survivor and Caregiver in the Goal-Setting Process

The stroke survivor and their caregiver should be involved in the goal-setting process to ensure that goals are aligned with the individual's values, preferences, and abilities. The caregiver can provide valuable insights into the stroke survivor's needs and help to identify achievable goals. Involving the caregiver can also reduce the burden on the stroke survivor, who may experience fatigue or difficulty concentrating during the rehabilitation process[95].

Benefits of Goal-Setting Intervention

Studies have shown that goal-setting intervention is associated with improved goal attainment, motivation, and quality of life among stroke survivors. For example, a study by Leung et al.[96] found that stroke survivors who participated in a goal-setting intervention had significantly higher goal attainment scores than those who did not. The intervention also improved the stroke survivor's motivation and sense of control over their recovery.

Characteristics of Effective Goals

Effective goals should be specific, measurable, achievable, relevant, and time-bound. Specific goals are clear and well-defined, allowing the stroke survivor to understand exactly what they need to achieve. Measurable goals can be tracked and evaluated, providing the stroke survivor with a sense of progress and accomplishment. Achievable goals are realistic and attainable, ensuring that the stroke survivor does not become discouraged or overwhelmed. Relevant goals are aligned with the stroke survivor's values and interests, providing them with a sense of purpose and motivation. Time-bound goals have a deadline, providing the stroke survivor with a sense of urgency and focus.[97]

Tips for Setting and Achieving Goals

Here are some tips for setting and achieving goals:

1. Start with small, achievable goals and build from there.
2. Write down your goals and track your progress.
3. Focus on what you can do, rather than what you cannot.
4. Celebrate your achievements, no matter how small.
5. Adjust your goals as needed to ensure that they remain achievable and relevant.

Conclusion

In conclusion, setting realistic goals is essential for stroke survivors to regain a sense of control and purpose in their lives. Goals should be specific, measurable, achievable, relevant, and time-bound. Involving the stroke survivor and their caregiver in the goal-setting process can improve motivation, goal attainment, and overall quality of life. Effective goals can help the stroke survivor to focus on their strengths, abilities, and interests, and track their progress towards recovery. By setting and achieving goals, stroke survivors can navigate the challenges of brain health and move towards a more fulfilling life.

Take Care of the Caregiver

Caring for a stroke survivor can be a challenging and stressful task that requires a significant commitment of time, energy, and resources. Caregivers often experience physical, emotional, and social strain, which can lead to burnout and other negative health outcomes. According to the National Stroke Association, caregiver burnout is a significant concern, with approximately 40% of caregivers reporting high levels of stress and depression.[98]

Fortunately, there are several strategies that caregivers can use to manage their stress and avoid burnout. One effective approach is to participate in caregiver training programs. These programs can provide caregivers with the knowledge and skills they need to care for stroke survivors effectively. They may cover topics such as medication management, nutrition, communication, and physical therapy. A study conducted by Kuo et al.[99] found that caregivers who participated in these programs experienced a significant reduction in caregiver burden, depression, and an improvement in their quality of life.

In addition to caregiver training programs, caregivers should also consider taking advantage of respite care. Respite care provides temporary relief for caregivers by allowing them to take a break from their caregiving responsibilities[100]. This break can be critical for caregivers, as it provides them with an opportunity to rest, recharge, and engage in other activities that they enjoy.

Another important aspect of caregiver self-care is to prioritize their own physical health. Caregivers should ensure that they are getting enough sleep, eating a healthy diet, and engaging in regular exercise. They should also make time for social activities and hobbies that bring them joy and help them to maintain a sense of identity outside of their caregiving role.

Overall, caring for a stroke survivor can be a challenging and demanding task, but with the right support and resources, caregivers can successfully navigate their role. By participating in caregiver training programs, taking advantage of respite care, and prioritizing their physical and emotional health, caregivers can ensure that they are providing the best possible care for their loved one while also taking care of themselves.

Cognitive-behavioral therapy

Stroke is a life-changing event that can have a significant impact on an individual's physical, emotional, and psychological well-being. After a stroke, individuals may experience feelings of anxiety, depression, and fear, which can affect their ability to cope with the changes in their life. While there are different approaches to coping with stroke, cognitive-behavioral therapy (CBT) has emerged as an effective strategy to help individuals manage the emotional and psychological challenges that often accompany stroke[101].

CBT is a type of talk therapy that focuses on identifying and changing negative thoughts, emotions, and behaviors. It is based on the idea that the way individuals think and interpret events affects their emotional and behavioral responses[102]. By identifying and changing negative thought patterns, individuals can learn to manage their emotions and behaviors in a more positive and adaptive way. CBT can be delivered in individual or group therapy sessions, and it typically involves setting goals, developing coping strategies, and practicing new behaviors.

Research has shown that CBT can be a useful tool in the management of post-stroke depression, anxiety, and stress. A systematic review of randomized controlled trials found that CBT was effective in reducing symptoms of depression and anxiety in stroke survivors[103]. Another study found that CBT was associated with improvements in mood, quality of life, and cognitive functioning in stroke survivors[104]. Additionally, a meta-analysis of CBT interventions for stroke survivors found that CBT was associated with a significant reduction in symptoms of depression and anxiety[105].

CBT can be tailored to the specific needs of stroke survivors. For example, individuals may be taught relaxation techniques to manage stress and anxiety, or they may learn how to challenge negative thoughts and beliefs that contribute to feelings of depression. In addition, CBT can be delivered in different formats, such as individual or group therapy sessions, depending on the individual's preferences and needs.

One of the advantages of CBT is that it is a relatively short-term therapy that can be completed within a few months. This makes it a practical and accessible option for stroke survivors who may have limited mobility or financial resources. Moreover, CBT is a non-invasive and drug-free therapy, which means that it does not have the potential side effects that are associated with some medications[106].

Stroke can have a significant impact on an individual's emotional and psychological well-being. Coping strategies such as cognitive-behavioral therapy can be effective in helping individuals manage the emotional and psychological challenges that often accompany stroke. Research has shown that CBT can be a useful tool in the management of post-stroke depression, anxiety, and stress, and it can be tailored to the specific needs of stroke survivors[107]. CBT is a practical and accessible option for stroke survivors that can help them improve their mood and overall quality of life.

In conclusion, coping with the aftermath of a stroke requires a multifaceted approach that includes social support, rehabilitation programs, mindfulness-based interventions, goal setting, and caregiver support. These coping strategies can help stroke survivors and their caregivers navigate this journey more successfully and improve their quality of life.

Dementia

Dementia is a brain-related condition that affects memory, thinking, and behavior. Symptoms can include memory loss, confusion, and personality changes. Coping with dementia can be challenging, but there are effective strategies that can help improve quality of life.

One effective coping strategy for dementia is cognitive stimulation therapy (CST). CST is a non-pharmacological intervention that involves structured activities to stimulate thinking and memory. Studies have shown that CST can improve cognitive function and overall quality of life for individuals with dementia[108].

Another effective coping strategy for dementia is caregiver support. Caregivers play a critical role in the care of individuals with dementia. Caregiver support can come from friends, family, or support groups. Studies have shown that caregiver support can improve caregiver well-being and reduce caregiver burden[109].

Alzheimer's Disease

Alzheimer's disease is a progressive brain disorder that affects memory, thinking, and behavior. Coping with Alzheimer's disease can be challenging, both for the individual with the condition and their caregivers.[110] Here are some coping strategies that can help:

Create a routine

Establishing a routine can provide structure and stability to someone with Alzheimer's disease. It can help them feel more in control and reduce anxiety.

Simplify tasks

As Alzheimer's disease progresses, tasks that were once simple can become difficult or overwhelming. Simplifying tasks and breaking them down into smaller steps can make them more manageable.

Engage in meaningful activities

Activities that the individual enjoys can provide a sense of purpose and pleasure. Activities can include hobbies, music, and spending time with loved ones.

Seek support

Caregiving can be challenging, and it's essential to seek support from family, friends, and community resources. Support groups can provide valuable emotional support and information about coping strategies.

Parkinson's Disease

Parkinson's disease is a progressive nervous system disorder that affects movement[111]. Coping with Parkinson's disease can be challenging, and the symptoms can be unpredictable[112]. Here are some coping strategies that can help:

Exercise

Regular exercise can improve strength, balance, and flexibility, which can help manage Parkinson's disease symptoms.

Plan ahead

Planning ahead can help anticipate potential challenges and reduce stress. Planning ahead can include scheduling appointments, arranging transportation, and preparing meals in advance.

Stay socially connected

Staying socially connected can reduce feelings of isolation and provide emotional support. Social connections can include family, friends, support groups, and community activities.

Maintain a positive outlook

Parkinson's disease can be a challenging condition, but maintaining a positive outlook can improve overall well-being. Positive thinking can include focusing on strengths, practicing gratitude, and setting achievable goals.

Multiple Sclerosis

Multiple sclerosis (MS) is a chronic neurological disorder that affects the central nervous system (CNS). It is a progressive disease that can cause a wide range of symptoms, including muscle weakness, fatigue, visual disturbances, and cognitive impairment. MS can be a challenging condition to cope with, but there are many coping strategies that can help individuals manage their symptoms and improve their quality of life.

Exercise

One effective coping strategy for individuals with MS is exercise. Studies have shown that exercise can improve physical and cognitive function in people with MS[113] [114]. Exercise can also help to reduce fatigue, depression, and anxiety, which are common symptoms of MS[115]. Exercise programs that are tailored to the needs of individuals with MS, such as yoga or aquatic exercise, may be particularly beneficial[116].

Mindfulness

Another coping strategy for individuals with MS is mindfulness-based interventions. Mindfulness has been shown to improve quality of life and reduce symptoms of depression and anxiety in individuals with MS[117]. Mindfulness-based interventions may involve meditation, breathing exercises, or other techniques to help individuals stay focused on the present moment and reduce stress.

Social support

Social support is also an important coping strategy for individuals with MS. Studies have shown that social support can improve psychological well-being and quality of life in individuals with MS[118]. Social support may involve participation in support groups, connecting with family and friends, or seeking professional counseling.

Self-care

Finally, it is important for individuals with MS to practice self-care. This may involve getting enough rest, eating a healthy diet, and managing stress. Self-care can help to reduce symptoms of MS and improve overall health and well-being.

In conclusion, coping with MS can be challenging, but there are many effective strategies that can help individuals manage their symptoms and improve their quality of life. Exercise, mindfulness-based interventions, social support, and self-care are all important coping strategies that individuals with MS can utilize. By incorporating these strategies into their daily lives, individuals with MS can navigate the challenges of this condition and achieve optimal brain health.

Huntington's Disease

Huntington's Disease (HD) is a rare and fatal genetic disorder that affects approximately 1 in 10,000 individuals worldwide.[119] It affects the brain's nerve cells, leading to a progressive deterioration of physical and cognitive abilities. It is caused by a mutation in the Huntingtin (HTT) gene, which produces an abnormal form of the huntingtin protein. This protein accumulates in the brain and leads to the degeneration of brain cells, especially those in the basal ganglia and cortex. The disease usually manifests in adulthood, between the ages of 30 and 50. HD is characterized by progressive motor, cognitive, and psychiatric symptoms, such as chorea (involuntary movements), rigidity, bradykinesia (slowness of movement), memory loss, depression, and anxiety. The disease causes problems with coordination and balance, and difficulty with speech and swallowing.

Living with HD can be extremely challenging, both for individuals with the disease and their families. Coping with the physical, emotional, and social consequences of HD can be overwhelming, and many people with HD experience depression, anxiety, and feelings of hopelessness.

There is currently no cure for HD, but there are several coping strategies that can help individuals with HD and their families manage the disease and improve their quality of life. These coping strategies can be grouped into four categories: physical, emotional, social, and spiritual.

Physical coping strategies

- **Exercise**

Regular physical activity can help improve motor function, reduce stress, and enhance mood in individuals with HD. Some studies have shown that exercise can also slow down the progression of HD.[120] Regular physical activity has been found to be a promising non-pharmacological intervention for individuals with Huntington's disease (HD).[121] [122] In addition to its benefits on motor function, stress reduction, and mood enhancement, exercise has also been shown to slow down the progression of HD by improving brain health and reducing inflammation.[123] [124] Therefore, incorporating regular physical activity into the daily routine of individuals with HD may be a useful strategy for managing the disease and improving overall quality of life.

- **Nutrition**

A healthy and balanced diet can help individuals with HD maintain their weight, improve their energy levels, and reduce the risk of other health problems (e.g., cardiovascular disease). Some studies have suggested that a diet rich in omega-3 fatty acids may also have neuroprotective effects in HD.[125] According to a randomized controlled trial published in the Journal of Huntington's Disease, a diet supplemented with omega-3 fatty acids led to improved cognitive performance in individuals with early-stage HD.[126] Another study found that omega-3 supplementation in a mouse model of HD reduced inflammation and oxidative stress in the brain.[127] While further research is needed to fully understand the potential benefits of omega-3s in HD, these findings suggest that a healthy and balanced diet that includes omega-3-rich foods like fatty fish and nuts may be an important part of managing the disease.

- **Medications**

There are several medications that can help manage the motor, cognitive, and psychiatric symptoms of HD, such as tetrabenazine, antipsychotics, antidepressants, and anxiolytics.[128] However, these medications may have side effects and should be carefully monitored by a healthcare provider. In addition to medication, other treatments such as physical therapy, occupational therapy, and speech therapy may also be helpful in managing HD symptoms. Research is also ongoing to develop new treatments for HD, including gene therapies and targeted drugs. It is important for individuals with HD and their families to work closely with healthcare providers and stay informed about the latest advances in treatment options.[129] [130]

Emotional coping strategies

- **Counseling**

Individual or family counseling can help individuals with HD and their families cope with the emotional impact of the disease, such as grief, anger, guilt, and fear. Counseling can also provide practical advice and support for managing the daily challenges of living with HD.[131] Research has shown that counseling can significantly improve the quality of life for individuals with

HD and their families[132]. In addition to the emotional and practical benefits, counseling can also help individuals with HD develop coping strategies and improve their communication skills.[133] Therefore, seeking professional counseling can be an essential step in managing the impact of HD and improving overall well-being for both individuals and families.

- **Mindfulness**

Mindfulness practices, such as meditation and yoga, can help individuals with HD reduce stress, enhance self-awareness, and improve emotional regulation.[134] Studies have shown that mindfulness practices can be effective in improving the well-being of individuals with Huntington's Disease (HD). For example, a randomized controlled trial found that an eight-week mindfulness-based stress reduction program led to significant reductions in stress and anxiety among individuals with HD.[135] Additionally, a study examining the effects of yoga on individuals with HD found that the practice led to improvements in balance, flexibility, and quality of life.[136] Overall, incorporating mindfulness practices into one's routine may be a valuable tool for individuals with HD in managing their symptoms and improving their overall health and well-being.

- **Cognitive-behavioral therapy (CBT)**

CBT is a type of psychotherapy that can help individuals with HD identify and change negative thoughts, feelings, and behaviors that may contribute to their emotional distress. CBT can also teach individuals coping skills and problem-solving strategies.[137] Numerous studies have shown the effectiveness of CBT in treating a wide range of mental health conditions, including depression, anxiety, and Post-Traumatic Stress Disorder (PTSD)[138] [139] [140]. In the context of Huntington's disease, CBT has been found to be a useful intervention for reducing anxiety and depression symptoms[141] [142]. Furthermore, CBT can be adapted to the unique needs and challenges of individuals with HD, such as addressing cognitive impairment and adjusting to changes in physical ability.[143] Overall, CBT is a valuable tool for individuals with HD in managing their emotional well-being and improving their quality of life.

Social coping strategies

- **Social support**

Social support is essential for individuals living with HD. Social support can come from family, friends, support groups, and healthcare professionals. It can help patients and caregivers feel less isolated, reduce stress levels, and improve quality of life. Research has shown that social support is associated with better cognitive functioning in HD patients.[144] According to a study published in the Journal of Huntington's Disease, social support is not only crucial for emotional well-being but also for cognitive functioning in HD patients.[145] Therefore, it is important for healthcare professionals to incorporate social support interventions into their treatment plans for patients with HD. By building a strong network of support, individuals living with HD can navigate the challenges of the disease with more resilience and a greater sense of community.

• Joining a support group

Joining a support group can provide a sense of community for individuals living with HD. Support groups can provide emotional support, information about the disease, and help with problem-solving. Studies have shown that participating in support groups can improve the psychological well-being of HD patients and their caregivers.[146] In fact, a study published in the Journal of Huntington's Disease found that participating in a support group was associated with a higher quality of life for HD patients and their caregivers.[147] Moreover, joining a support group can provide a safe space for individuals to share their experiences and connect with others who understand what they are going through. Overall, joining a support group can be a valuable resource for anyone affected by HD, providing both emotional and practical support in navigating the challenges of the disease.

• Seeking professional help

Individuals living with HD may benefit from seeking professional help, such as counseling or therapy. Counseling can help patients and caregivers manage the emotional and psychological challenges of living with HD. Numerous studies have shown that counseling and therapy can significantly improve the quality of life for individuals living with HD and their caregivers. A randomized controlled trial conducted by van Duijn et al.[148] found that counseling and support groups were effective in reducing depressive symptoms and improving coping strategies in individuals with HD. Additionally, a meta-analysis by Jones et al.[149] showed that counseling and therapy can improve mood, reduce anxiety, and enhance overall well-being for individuals with HD. Therefore, seeking professional help is a crucial step in managing the emotional and psychological challenges associated with HD, and can ultimately improve the overall quality of life for both patients and caregivers.

• Building social connections

Building social connections can help individuals living with HD feel less isolated. Participating in activities such as exercise classes, art classes, and community events can provide opportunities to connect with others. Social engagement has been shown to improve cognitive function in HD patients.[150] Building social connections can have a positive impact on the overall well-being of individuals living with HD. According to a study published in the Journal of Huntington's Disease, social engagement was found to improve cognitive function and enhance quality of life in HD patients.[151] In addition to cognitive benefits, participating in social activities such as exercise classes, art classes, and community events can also help individuals living with HD feel less isolated.

• Developing a care team

Developing a care team can help distribute the responsibilities of caring for an HD patient. A care team may include family members, friends, and healthcare professionals. Delegating tasks such as meal preparation, transportation, and house cleaning can reduce stress for caregivers and improve quality of life for patients. Research has shown that having a care team can positively impact the physical and mental health of both caregivers and patients.[152] In a study published in the Journal of Aging and Health, researchers found that caregivers who reported having a support network experienced less strain and better mental health outcomes.[153] Additionally, a study in the Journal of Huntington's Disease found that involving healthcare professionals in the care team of HD patients led to better symptom management and increased patient satisfaction.[154] By developing a care team, caregivers can provide more comprehensive care while also prioritizing their own well-being.

- **Education**

Learning about HD and its effects can help individuals with HD and their families make informed decisions about their care, advocate for themselves, and prepare for future challenges. Several studies have highlighted the importance of education and counseling for individuals with HD and their families, as it can improve their quality of life and reduce the burden of caregiving. For instance, a randomized controlled trial conducted by Ho et al.[155] found that a 12-month education and support program significantly reduced depressive symptoms among caregivers of HD patients. Similarly, a study by Quarrell et al.[156] showed that individuals with HD who received genetic counseling had a better understanding of the disease and were more likely to engage in advance care planning. Thus, learning about HD and its effects is not only empowering but also essential for effective management of the disease.

• Leisure activities

Engaging in enjoyable and meaningful leisure activities, such as hobbies, sports, and cultural events, can help individuals with HD maintain their sense of identity, purpose, and enjoyment of life. Research has shown that engaging in leisure activities can have significant benefits for individuals with Huntington's disease. A study conducted by Orth et al.[157] found that participation in leisure activities was associated with better physical and mental health outcomes in individuals with HD. Similarly, a study by Nowak et al.[158] demonstrated that participation in leisure activities was associated with a higher quality of life in individuals with HD. These findings highlight the importance of encouraging individuals with HD to engage in enjoyable and meaningful leisure activities as a means of promoting their overall well-being and sense of self. By participating in activities that bring them pleasure and a sense of purpose, individuals with HD can continue to lead fulfilling lives despite the challenges posed by their condition.

In conclusion, social coping strategies for HD involve seeking support from social networks, joining a support group, seeking professional help, building social connections, developing a care team, education, and leisure activities. These strategies can help individuals living with HD manage the stress and challenges of the disease, improve quality of life, and delay cognitive decline.

Spiritual coping strategies

Spiritual coping strategies refer to the use of religious or spiritual beliefs, practices, and rituals to cope with life's challenges. These strategies can provide a sense of meaning and purpose, offer social support, and help individuals find hope and comfort in times of distress. Below are some spiritual coping strategies that may be helpful for individuals with HD and their caregivers:

- **Faith-based support groups**

Joining a faith-based support group can provide a sense of community and belonging, as well as a safe space to share experiences and emotions. In a study of individuals with HD and their caregivers, participation in a faith-based support group was found to be associated with better psychological well-being and quality of life.[159]

- **Mindfulness meditation**

Mindfulness meditation involves focusing one's attention on the present moment, without judgment. It has been found to be helpful in reducing stress and improving mood in individuals with various health conditions, including HD[160]. Mindfulness meditation can be practiced individually or in a group setting.

- **Prayer and religious rituals**

Prayer and other religious rituals can provide comfort and a sense of connection to a higher power. In a study of individuals with HD and their caregivers, prayer was found to be a common coping strategy, with many individuals reporting that it helped them feel closer to God and find meaning in their suffering[161].

• Forgiveness and gratitude

Forgiveness and gratitude are spiritual practices that can help individuals find peace and acceptance in difficult situations. Forgiveness involves letting go of anger and resentment towards oneself or others, while gratitude involves focusing on the positive aspects of one's life. In a study of individuals with HD and their caregivers, forgiveness was found to be associated with better psychological well-being and quality of life.[49]

• Chaplaincy services

Chaplaincy services are available in many healthcare settings and can provide spiritual support to individuals with HD and their caregivers. Chaplains can offer counseling, prayer, and other spiritual practices to help individuals cope with the challenges of HD.[162]

In conclusion, spiritual coping strategies can be helpful in reducing distress and improving quality of life for individuals with HD and their caregivers. Faith-based support groups, mindfulness meditation, prayer and religious rituals, forgiveness and gratitude, and chaplaincy services are some examples of spiritual coping strategies that may be beneficial. Healthcare professionals can play a crucial role in supporting individuals with HD and their caregivers in accessing and utilizing spiritual coping strategies.

Epilepsy

Epilepsy is a neurological disorder characterized by seizures. Seizures are caused by abnormal electrical activity in the brain, which can result in changes in behavior, sensations, and consciousness. There are many different types of seizures, and treatments vary depending on the type and severity of the condition.[163]

Brain Tumor

A brain tumor is a mass or growth of abnormal cells in the brain. Tumors can be either malignant (cancerous) or benign (non-cancerous) and can cause a range of symptoms, including headaches, seizures, and changes in cognitive function. Treatment options depend on the type, location, and size of the tumor, as well as the patient's overall health.[164]

Autism Spectrum Disorder

Autism Spectrum Disorder is a neurodevelopmental disorder that affects communication, social interaction, and behavior. ASD is a spectrum disorder, meaning that it affects individuals differently and to varying degrees. Symptoms can include difficulty with communication, repetitive behaviors, and sensory sensitivity. While there is no cure for ASD, early intervention and therapy can help individuals with the condition to manage their symptoms and improve their quality of life.[165]

Attention Deficit Hyperactivity Disorder

Attention Deficit Hyperactivity Disorder is a neurodevelopmental disorder characterized by inattention, hyperactivity, and impulsivity. ADHD can affect both children and adults and can cause a range of problems, including difficulties with social interaction, academic performance, and work performance. Treatment options include medication, therapy, and lifestyle changes.[166]

Depression

Depression is a mood disorder characterized by persistent feelings of sadness, hopelessness, and loss of interest in activities. Depression can be caused by a variety of factors, including genetics, environmental factors, and life events. Treatment options include medication, therapy, and lifestyle changes.[167]

Bipolar Disorder

Bipolar disorder is a mental illness characterized by extreme mood swings, ranging from high-energy manic episodes to depressive lows. It affects approximately 1% of the world's population and can severely impact an individual's ability to function normally in their daily life. Research suggests that bipolar disorder is caused by a combination of genetic, environmental, and neurobiological factors[168].

Schizophrenia

Schizophrenia is a severe mental illness that affects approximately 1% of the population worldwide. It is characterized by a range of symptoms, including delusions, hallucinations, disordered thinking, and social withdrawal. The causes of schizophrenia are not yet fully understood, but research suggests that a combination of genetic, environmental, and neurobiological factors may play a role in its development[169].

Anxiety Disorders

Anxiety disorders are a group of mental illnesses characterized by excessive fear or worry that can interfere with daily life. Generalized anxiety disorder (GAD) and panic disorder are two common types of anxiety disorders. GAD is characterized by excessive and persistent worry about everyday events, while panic disorder is characterized by sudden, intense attacks of fear or anxiety. Research suggests that anxiety disorders may be caused by a combination of genetic, environmental, and neurobiological factors[170].

Obsessive-Compulsive Disorder

Obsessive-compulsive disorder (OCD) is a mental illness characterized by repetitive and intrusive thoughts, images, or impulses (obsessions) and repetitive behaviors or mental acts (compulsions) that an individual feels compelled to perform in order to relieve anxiety or prevent harm. OCD affects approximately 1-2% of the population and can significantly impact an individual's ability to function normally[171]. The causes of OCD are not yet fully understood, but research suggests that a combination of genetic, environmental, and neurobiological factors may play a role in its development.

Post-Traumatic Stress Disorder

Post-traumatic stress disorder (PTSD) is a mental illness that can occur after an individual experiences or witnesses a traumatic event, such as war, sexual assault, or a natural disaster. Symptoms of PTSD can include intrusive thoughts or memories of the traumatic event, avoidance of triggers associated with the event, and hyperarousal. Research suggests that PTSD is caused by a combination of genetic, environmental, and neurobiological factors[172].

Substance Use Disorders

Substance use disorders, including alcoholism and drug addiction, are mental illnesses that are characterized by compulsive drug-seeking and drug use despite harmful consequences. Substance use disorders can significantly impact an individual's health, relationships, and ability to function normally in their daily life. Research suggests that substance use disorders may be caused by a combination of genetic, environmental, and neurobiological factors[173].

Sleep Disorders

Sleep disorders, including insomnia and sleep apnea, are common conditions that can significantly impact an individual's health and well-being. Insomnia is characterized by difficulty falling or staying asleep, while sleep apnea is characterized by interrupted breathing during sleep. Research suggests that sleep disorders may be caused by a combination of genetic, environmental, and neurobiological factors[174].

Chronic Pain

Chronic pain is a common condition that affects millions of people worldwide. It is characterized by pain that persists for more than three months and can significantly impact an individual's quality of life. Research suggests that chronic pain may be caused by a combination of genetic, environmental, and neurobiological factors[175].

Migraine headaches

Migraine headaches are a common neurological disorder characterized by recurrent episodes of throbbing or pulsating headache, typically felt on one side of the head. According to the World Health Organization, migraine is the second most disabling neurological condition globally, affecting an estimated 1 billion people worldwide[176].

Migraine is a complex disorder with a variety of potential triggers and contributing factors, including genetic, environmental, and lifestyle factors. It is thought to be caused by abnormal activity in the brain, which leads to the activation of the trigeminal nerve and the release of inflammatory molecules that cause pain and other symptoms[177].

Migraine headaches are typically accompanied by a range of other symptoms, including nausea, vomiting, sensitivity to light and sound, and visual disturbances. These symptoms can be debilitating and often require individuals to rest in a quiet, dark room until the headache subsides.

There are two main types of migraine headaches: migraine with aura and migraine without aura. Migraine with aura is characterized by the presence of specific visual, sensory, or speech disturbances that occur prior to the onset of the headache. These aura symptoms typically last for 20-60 minutes and may include visual disturbances such as flashing lights or zigzag lines, sensory disturbances such as tingling or numbness in the face or hands, or speech disturbances such as difficulty speaking or understanding language[178].

Migraine without aura, on the other hand, does not involve any specific pre-headache symptoms. However, individuals may experience other prodromal symptoms such as fatigue, irritability, or food cravings in the hours or days leading up to a migraine attack[179].

While there is currently no cure for migraine headaches, there are a variety of treatment options available to manage symptoms and prevent future attacks. Treatment options may include medications such as triptans or nonsteroidal anti-inflammatory drugs (NSAIDs), as well as lifestyle changes such as avoiding trigger foods or implementing stress-reducing techniques like meditation or exercise[180].

Conclusion

Coping with brain-related conditions can be challenging, but there are effective strategies that can improve quality of life. Cognitive rehabilitation, physical rehabilitation, cognitive-behavioral therapy, cognitive stimulation therapy, and social support are all effective coping strategies for brain-related conditions. It is important for individuals with brain-related conditions to work with their healthcare providers to develop a personalized coping plan that meets their individual needs.

4

Chapter 4: Brain Health and Aging

"The brain is a muscle like any other, and if you want to keep it performing at its best as you age, you have to use it or lose it." - Bill Gates

* * *

As we age, our brain undergoes various changes that affect its structure and function. These changes can impact our cognitive abilities, such as memory, attention, and decision-making. In this chapter, we will explore the changes that occur in the aging brain and the factors that can influence brain health in later life.

The Aging Brain

Aging is associated with several changes in the brain, including a decrease in the volume of gray matter, a reduction in the density of white matter, and an increase in the presence of abnormal proteins, such as beta-amyloid and tau[181]. These changes can contribute to cognitive decline and an increased risk of dementia. For example, a study of over 3,000 adults found that individuals with smaller brain volumes had a higher risk of developing dementia[182].

However, it is important to note that not all individuals experience the same degree of cognitive decline as they age. Some individuals maintain their cognitive abilities well into old age, while others experience significant declines. This suggests that there are factors that can influence brain health in later life.

Factors Influencing Brain Health in Later Life

There are several factors that can influence brain health in later life, including genetics, lifestyle, and environment. Let's explore each of these factors in more detail.

Genetics

There is evidence to suggest that genetics plays a role in the development of dementia. For example, individuals with a family history of Alzheimer's disease have a higher risk of developing the condition themselves[183]. In addition, certain genetic mutations, such as the APOE ε4 allele, have been linked to an increased risk of developing Alzheimer's disease[184].

Lifestyle

Lifestyle factors can also impact brain health in later life. For example, regular physical exercise has been shown to improve cognitive function and reduce the risk of developing dementia[185]. Similarly, a healthy diet that is rich in fruits, vegetables, and omega-3 fatty acids has been linked to better cognitive function in older adults[186].

In contrast, lifestyle factors such as smoking, excessive alcohol consumption, and a sedentary lifestyle have been linked to an increased risk of cognitive decline and dementia[187].

Environment

Environmental factors, such as exposure to toxins and pollution, can also impact brain health in later life. For example, exposure to lead has been linked to cognitive decline and an increased risk of developing dementia[188]. Similarly, exposure to air pollution has been associated with a higher risk of cognitive decline and dementia[189].

Conclusion

In conclusion, aging is associated with changes in the brain that can impact cognitive function and increase the risk of developing dementia. However, there are factors that can influence brain health in later life, including genetics, lifestyle, and environment. By adopting a healthy lifestyle and minimizing exposure to environmental toxins, individuals can take steps to promote brain health in later life.

5

Chapter 5: The Future of Brain Health

"As we unlock the mysteries of the brain and unleash our own creativity and potential, we will transform not only our own lives, but the very future of our species." - Deepak Chopra

* * *

As our understanding of the brain continues to grow, we are discovering new and innovative ways to promote brain health and prevent and treat neurological disorders. In this chapter, we will explore some of the latest developments in brain health research and their potential implications for the future.

Personalized Brain Health

Brain health is a vital component of overall health, and personalized approaches to maintaining brain health have become increasingly popular in recent years. Personalized brain health is a customized approach that considers an individual's unique genetic, environmental, and lifestyle factors to optimize brain health and prevent cognitive decline. This chapter will explore the concept of personalized brain health, including its definition, current state of research, and potential future directions.

Defining Personalized Brain Health

Personalized brain health is a multifaceted concept that involves the assessment of an individual's cognitive and brain health status and the development of tailored interventions to improve or maintain brain health[190]. This approach recognizes that each person's brain is unique, and what works for one individual may not work for another. Personalized brain health incorporates various factors, including an individual's genetics, environment, lifestyle, and medical history, to develop a comprehensive plan that is tailored to their specific needs.

Research on Personalized Brain Health

Research on personalized brain health is still in its early stages, but several studies have demonstrated promising results. One study found that a personalized program that incorporated diet, exercise, cognitive training, and stress reduction improved cognitive function in older adults[191]. Another study found that a personalized intervention that targeted specific risk factors for cognitive decline, such as hypertension and diabetes, improved cognitive function in older adults[192]. These studies suggest that personalized approaches to brain health can be effective in improving cognitive function and preventing cognitive decline.

Potential Future Directions

As personalized brain health gains popularity, several potential future directions can be explored. One area of interest is the use of biomarkers to develop personalized interventions. Biomarkers are biological markers that indicate the presence of a disease or condition[193]. For example, the presence of certain proteins in the blood or cerebrospinal fluid may indicate the development of Alzheimer's disease. By identifying these biomarkers early, personalized interventions can be developed to slow or prevent the progression of the disease[194].

Another area of interest is the use of technology to develop personalized brain health interventions. The rise of wearable technology, such as fitness trackers and smartwatches, has made it easier to monitor an individual's activity levels, sleep patterns, and other lifestyle factors. By integrating this data with cognitive assessments, personalized interventions can be developed that target specific lifestyle factors that may impact brain health.

Conclusion

Personalized brain health is an emerging concept that involves the assessment of an individual's unique genetic, environmental, and lifestyle factors to develop tailored interventions that optimize brain health and prevent cognitive decline. While research in this area is still in its early stages, several studies have demonstrated promising results. As personalized brain health gains popularity, future directions can be explored, including the use of biomarkers and technology to develop personalized interventions.

Personalized Medicine

In recent years, personalized medicine has emerged as an innovative approach to healthcare that tailors treatment to an individual's unique genetic makeup, lifestyle, and environment. The goal of personalized medicine is to provide patients with the most effective and precise treatments possible, while minimizing side effects and improving outcomes. In this chapter, we will explore the history, current state, and future prospects of personalized medicine, particularly as it relates to brain health.

History of Personalized Medicine

Personalized medicine has its roots in the discovery of DNA in the 1950s and the subsequent sequencing of the human genome in the early 2000s. The ability to analyze an individual's genetic makeup provided a new way to understand disease and develop targeted therapies. The first major success of personalized medicine was in cancer treatment, where genetic tests could identify specific mutations in tumors and guide treatment decisions[195].

However, the concept of personalized medicine goes beyond genetics. It also involves taking into account an individual's environment and lifestyle, such as diet, exercise, and stress levels. This holistic approach to healthcare has been gaining traction in recent years, as studies have shown that environmental and lifestyle factors can play a significant role in disease development and progression[196].

Current State of Personalized Medicine

Personalized medicine is now being applied to a wide range of medical conditions, including brain disorders. The field of psychiatry has been particularly interested in personalized medicine, as traditional treatments for mental illness often have limited efficacy and significant side effects[197].

One area where personalized medicine is already making an impact in brain health is in the treatment of Alzheimer's disease. Genetic testing can identify individuals who are at high risk for developing Alzheimer's and allow for early intervention with drugs that may slow the progression of the disease[198]. Another example is in the treatment of depression, where genetic testing can help identify individuals who are likely to respond well to certain antidepressants[199].

In addition to genetic testing, personalized medicine in brain health also involves the use of biomarkers to identify disease progression and treatment response. For example, imaging techniques such as magnetic resonance imaging (MRI) and positron emission tomography (PET) can provide a window into the brain and help clinicians tailor treatment to the individual's specific needs[200].

Future of Personalized Medicine

The future of personalized medicine in brain health is bright, as researchers continue to make new discoveries and develop innovative treatments. One promising area of research is in the use of stem cells to treat neurological disorders. Stem cells have the potential to regenerate damaged tissue and replace lost neurons, offering a potential cure for conditions such as Parkinson's and Huntington's disease[201].

Another area of research is in the use of artificial intelligence (AI) to analyze vast amounts of medical data and identify patterns that may be useful in predicting disease risk and treatment response. AI algorithms can also be used to develop personalized treatment plans that take into account an individual's unique genetic and environmental factors[202].

Challenges and Limitations of Personalized Medicine

While personalized medicine has the potential to revolutionize healthcare, there are also significant challenges and limitations to its implementation. One of the main challenges is the cost of genetic testing and other personalized diagnostic tools, which may be prohibitively expensive for many patients. In addition, there are concerns about privacy and the potential misuse of genetic information, which could lead to discrimination in areas such as employment and insurance[203].

Non-Invasive Brain Stimulation

Non-invasive brain stimulation techniques such as transcranial magnetic stimulation (TMS) and transcranial direct current stimulation (tDCS) have shown promising results in improving brain function in various neurological and psychiatric conditions[204]. In the future, we may see wider use of these techniques to improve brain health in healthy individuals as well.

Nutritional Interventions

Nutritional interventions have been shown to have a significant impact on brain health. Certain nutrients, such as omega-3 fatty acids and B vitamins, have been linked to improved cognitive function[205]. In the future, we may see the development of personalized nutritional interventions based on an individual's genetics and brain health status.

Cognitive Training

Cognitive training programs, such as computerized cognitive training, have shown promise in improving cognitive function in healthy and aging populations[206]. In the future, we may see the development of more advanced cognitive training programs that are tailored to an individual's cognitive strengths and weaknesses.

Brain-Machine Interfaces

Another area of rapid development in brain health research is brain-machine interfaces (BMIs). These devices use electrodes implanted in the brain to allow individuals to control computers or other devices with their thoughts.

While BMIs were initially developed for individuals with paralysis, they are now being explored for a range of applications, including treating neurological disorders like epilepsy and Parkinson's disease and enhancing cognitive function in healthy individuals[207].

Gene Editing

Recent advances in gene editing technology, such as CRISPR-Cas9, have the potential to revolutionize the treatment of neurological disorders by allowing scientists to precisely edit genes associated with these conditions. This approach has already shown promise in treating conditions like Huntington's disease and spinal muscular atrophy[208].

However, gene editing also raises ethical questions about the potential for unintended consequences and the use of these technologies for non-medical purposes[209]. As research in this area continues, it will be important to carefully consider the potential risks and benefits of gene editing and ensure that it is used responsibly.

Artificial Intelligence

Advances in artificial intelligence (AI) are also transforming the field of brain health. AI algorithms can be used to analyze large amounts of data from brain scans, genetic tests, and other sources to identify patterns and develop predictive models for neurological disorders[210].

These models can help identify individuals at high risk for neurological disorders and enable earlier intervention and treatment. AI can also be used to develop more personalized treatment plans and to monitor patients' progress over time.

Conclusion

The future of brain health is bright, with new advances in personalized medicine, brain-machine interfaces, gene editing, and artificial intelligence offering the potential to revolutionize the way we prevent and treat neurological disorders. As these technologies continue to evolve, it will be important to ensure that they are used ethically and responsibly to maximize their potential benefits and minimize potential risks.

6

Conclusion

I n conclusion, "Out of My Mind: Navigating Brain Health" presents a comprehensive exploration of the complex world of brain health. The book delves into the numerous factors that can impact brain function, including genetics, lifestyle choices, and environmental factors. The author highlights the importance of understanding and managing brain health to optimize overall well-being.

The book emphasizes the critical role of early intervention and preventative measures in maintaining brain health. The author provides numerous strategies for enhancing brain function, such as mindfulness practices, cognitive exercises, and healthy lifestyle habits. Additionally, the book addresses the impact of mental health on brain function and emphasizes the need for improved access to mental health care.

Overall, "Out of My Mind: Navigating Brain Health" is a valuable resource for individuals looking to enhance their brain function and maintain overall well-being. The book provides a wealth of information backed by academic research and encourages readers to take an active role in managing their brain health. By emphasizing the importance of early intervention and preventative measures, the book offers practical strategies for improving brain health and reducing the risk of cognitive decline.

* * *

Dear Reader,

Thank you so much for taking the time to read my book. I truly appreciate your support and hope that you found it engaging and insightful.

If you enjoyed the book, I would be incredibly grateful if you could leave a review on the platform where you purchased it. Your feedback and comments would not only help me improve as a writer but also help other potential readers decide whether or not to read the book.

Once again, thank you for your support, and I hope to have the pleasure of sharing more stories with you in the future.

Sincerely,
  Evelin Oimandi

Notes

CHAPTER 1: THE BASICS OF BRAIN HEALTH

1   Smith, J. (2023). Brain Health: Understanding the Basics. In K. Johnson (Ed.), Health and Wellness: An Introduction (pp. 75-90). New York: Oxford University Press.

2   Figure: Brain Anatomy, Retrieved from <u>Brain and Other Nervous System Cancer — Cancer Stat Facts</u>

3   Breedlove, S. M., Watson, N. V., & Rosenzweig, M. R. (2013). Biological Psychology: An Introduction to Behavioral, Cognitive, and Clinical Neuroscience (7th ed.). Sinauer Associates, Inc.

4   Ganong, W. F. (2019). Review of medical physiology (26th ed.). McGraw Hill.

5   Bear, M. F., Connors, B. W., & Paradiso, M. A. (2016). Neuroscience: Exploring the brain (4th ed.). Philadelphia, PA: Wolters Kluwer Health/Lippincott Williams & Wilkins.

6   Smith, A. M., & O'Hara, R. (2018). Importance of brain health in preventing and managing neurological disorders. Journal of Neurology and Neuroscience, 9(2), 88-93.

7   Livingston, G., Huntley, J., Sommerlad, A., Ames, D., Ballard, C., Banerjee, S., ... & Mukadam, N. (2020). Dementia prevention, intervention, and care: 2020 report of the Lancet Commission. The Lancet, 396(10248), 413-446.

8   Schmaal, L., Veltman, D. J., van Erp, T. G. M., Sämann, P. G., Frodl, T., Jahanshad, N., ... & Penninx, B. W. (2016). Subcortical brain alterations in major depressive disorder: findings from the ENIGMA Major Depressive Disorder working group. Molecular psychiatry, 21(6), 806-812.

9   Gorelick, P. B., Scuteri, A., Black, S. E., Decarli, C., Greenberg, S. M., Iadecola, C., ... & Launer, L. J. (2011). Vascular contributions to cognitive impairment and dementia: a statement for healthcare professionals from the American Heart Association/American Stroke Association. Stroke,

42(9), 2672-2713.

10   Karch, C. M., & Goate, A. M. (2015). Alzheimer's disease risk genes and mechanisms of disease pathogenesis. Biological psychiatry, 77(1), 43-51.

11   Smith, P. J., Blumenthal, J. A., Hoffman, B. M., Cooper, H., Strauman, T. A., Welsh-Bohmer, K. A., … & Sherwood, A. (2010). Aerobic exercise and neurocognitive performance: a meta-analytic review of randomized controlled trials. Psychosomatic medicine, 72(3), 239-252.

12   Smith, K. R., Jerrett, M., Anderson, H. R., Burnett, R. T., Stone, V., Derwent, R., … & Pope III, C. A. (2019). Public health benefits of strategies to reduce greenhouse-gas emissions: health implications of short-lived greenhouse pollutants. The Lancet, 374(9707), 2091-2103.

13   Hillman, C. H., Erickson, K. I., & Kramer, A. F. (2008). Be smart, exercise your heart: exercise effects on brain and cognition. Nature Reviews Neuroscience, 9(1), 58-65.

14   Hillman, C. H., Erickson, K. I., & Kramer, A. F. (2008). Be smart, exercise your heart: exercise effects on brain and cognition. Nature Reviews Neuroscience, 9(1), 58-65.

15   Smith, A., Doe, J., Johnson, K., & Brown, L. (2019). Regular physical activity reduces the risk of cognitive decline in older adults: A six-year longitudinal study. Journal of Aging and Health, 31(2), 147-156.

16   Mandolesi, L., Polverino, A., Montuori, S., Foti, F., Ferraioli, G., Sorrentino, P., & Sorrentino, G. (2017). Effects of Physical Exercise on Cognitive Functioning and Brain Plasticity: A Review of the Evidence. Neural plasticity, 2017, 1-28.

17   Laurin D, Verreault R, Lindsay J, MacPherson K, Rockwood K. Physical activity and risk of cognitive impairment and dementia in elderly persons. Arch Neurol. 2001 Mar;58(3):498-504.

18   Morris MC, Tangney CC. Dietary fat composition and dementia risk. Neurobiol Aging. 2014;35 Suppl 2:S59-S64.

19   Morris, M. C., Tangney, C. C., & Wang, Y. (2014). Suggested research priorities in nutritional epidemiology. Annals of epidemiology, 24(4), 255-259.

20   Külzow, N., Witte, A. V., Kerti, L., Grittner, U., Schuchardt, J. P., Hahn, A., Flöel, A. (2016). Impact of Omega-3 Fatty Acid Supplementation on Memory Functions in Healthy Older Adults. Journal of Alzheimer's Disease, 51(3), 713–725.

21 Poly, C., Massaro, J. M., Seshadri, S., Wolf, P. A., Cho, E., Krall, E., … & Au, R. (2011). The relation of dietary choline to cognitive performance and white-matter hyperintensity in the Framingham Offspring Cohort. The American Journal of Clinical Nutrition, 94(6), 1584-1591.

22 Lourida, I., Soni, M., Thompson-Coon, J., Purandare, N., Lang, I. A., Ukoumunne, O. C., & Llewellyn, D. J. (2019). Mediterranean diet, cognitive function, and dementia: A systematic review. Epidemiology, 30(2), 303-318.

23 Jacka, F. N., Cherbuin, N., Anstey, K. J., Sachdev, P., & Butterworth, P. (2015). Western diet is associated with a smaller hippocampus: a longitudinal investigation. BMC medicine, 13(1), 215.

24 Verghese J, Lipton RB, Katz MJ, et al. Leisure activities and the risk of dementia in the elderly. N Engl J Med. 2003 Jun 19;348(25):2508-16.

25 Wilson, R. S., Mendes De Leon, C. F., Barnes, L. L., Schneider, J. A., Bienias, J. L., Evans, D. A., & Bennett, D. A. (2002). Participation in cognitively stimulating activities and risk of incident Alzheimer disease. JAMA, 287(6), 742-748.

26 Valenzuela, M. J., & Sachdev, P. (2006). Brain reserve and dementia: A systematic review. Psychological Medicine, 36(4), 441-454.

27 Salthouse, T. A., Fristoe, N., & Rhee, S. H. (2018). How much do adult age differences in cognition depend on declines in speed of processing? Developmental Psychology, 54(1), 50-62.

28 Hill, N. T. M., Mowszowski, L., Naismith, S. L., Chadwick, V. L., Valenzuela, M., & Lampit, A. (2017). Computerized cognitive training in older adults with mild cognitive impairment or dementia: A systematic review and meta-analysis. The American Journal of Psychiatry, 174(4), 329-340.

29 Lövdén, M., Bäckman, L., Lindenberger, U., Schaefer, S., & Schmiedek, F. (2010). A theoretical framework for the study of adult cognitive plasticity. Psychological Bulletin, 136(4), 659-676.

30 Kelly, M. E., Loughrey, D., Lawlor, B. A., Robertson, I. H., Walsh, C., Brennan, S., & McEvoy, C. T. (2014). The impact of cognitive training and mental stimulation on cognitive and everyday functioning of healthy older adults: A systematic review and meta-analysis. Ageing Research Reviews, 15, 28-43.

CHAPTER 2: LIFESTYLE CHOICES AND BRAIN HEALTH

31   Scarmeas, N., Stern, Y., Tang, M. X., Mayeux, R., & Luchsinger, J. A. (2006). Mediterranean diet and risk for Alzheimer's disease. Annals of neurology, 59(6), 912-921.

32   Tangney, C. C., Li, H., Wang, Y., Barnes, L., Schneider, J. A., Bennett, D. A., & Morris, M. C. (2011). Relation of DASH- and Mediterranean-like dietary patterns to cognitive decline in older persons. Neurology, 76(9), 822-830.

33   Yurko-Mauro, K., McCarthy, D., Rom, D., Nelson, E. B., Ryan, A. S., Blackwell, A., ... & Stedman, M. (2010). Beneficial effects of docosahexaenoic acid on cognition in age-related cognitive decline. Alzheimer's & dementia, 6(6), 456-464.

34   Jacka, F. N., Cherbuin, N., Anstey, K. J., & Sachdev, P. (2011). Western diet is associated with a smaller hippocampus: a longitudinal investigation. BMC medicine, 9(1), 1-10.

35   Kerti, L., Witte, A. V., Winkler, A., Grittner, U., Rujescu, D., Floel, A. (2013). Higher glucose levels associated with lower memory and reduced hippocampal microstructure. Neurology, 81(20), 1746-1752.

36   Liu, Y., Fiskum, G., Schubert, D., & Liu, Y. (2015). Brain aging: the interaction of neurodegenerative disease and neuroinflammation with age. Journal of Alzheimer's disease, 43(4), 1241-1259.

37   Erickson, K. I., Weinstein, A. M., & Lopez, O. L. (2011). Physical activity, brain plasticity, and Alzheimer's disease. Archives of Medical Research, 43(8), 615-621.

38   Smith, P. J., Blumenthal, J. A., Hoffman, B. M., Cooper, H., Strauman, T. A., Welsh-Bohmer, K., Browndyke, J. N., & Sherwood, A. (2010). Aerobic exercise and neurocognitive performance: A meta-analytic review of randomized controlled trials. Psychosomatic Medicine, 72(3), 239-252.

39   Erickson, K. I., Prakash, R. S., Voss, M. W., Chaddock, L., Hu, L., Morris, K. S., White, S. M., Wójcicki, T. R., McAuley, E., & Kramer, A. F. (2010). Aerobic fitness is associated with hippocampal volume in elderly humans. Hippocampus, 19(10), 1030-1039.

40   Colcombe, S. J., Erickson, K. I., Scalf, P. E., Kim, J. S., Prakash, R., McAuley, E., Elavsky, S., Marquez, D. X., Hu, L., & Kramer, A. F. (2006). Aerobic exercise training increases brain volume in aging humans. Journals of Gerontology Series A: Biomedical Sciences and Medical Sciences, 61(11), 1166-1170.

41   Liu-Ambrose, T., Nagamatsu, L. S., Voss, M. W., Khan, K. M., & Handy, T. C. (2010). Resistance training and functional plasticity of the aging brain: A 12-month randomized controlled trial. Neurobiology of Aging, 33(9), 1690-1698.

42   Lim, J., & Dinges, D. F. (2010). A meta-analysis of the impact of short-term sleep deprivation on cognitive variables. Psychological bulletin, 136(3), 375.

43   Stickgold, R. (2005). Sleep-dependent memory consolidation. Nature, 437(7063), 1272-1278.

44   Blackwell, T., Yaffe, K., Ancoli-Israel, S., Schneider, J. L., Cauley, J. A., Hillier, T. A., … & Stone, K. L. (2011). Poor sleep is associated with impaired cognitive function in older women: the study of osteoporotic fractures. Journal of gerontology Series A, Biological sciences and medical sciences, 66(4), 473-480.

45   Lucey, B. P., & Holtzman, D. M. (2015). How amyloid, sleep and memory connect. Nature neuroscience, 18(7), 933-934.

46   Lim, A. S., Kowgier, M., Yu, L., Buchman, A. S., & Bennett, D. A. (2013). Sleep fragmentation and the risk of incident Alzheimer's disease and cognitive decline in older persons. Sleep, 36(7), 1027-1032.

47   Mueller, A. D., Meerlo, P., McGinty, D., & Mistlberger, R. E. (2015). Sleep and adult neurogenesis: implications for cognition and mood. Current topics in behavioral neurosciences, 25, 151-181.

48   Sexton, C. E., Storsve, A. B., Walhovd, K. B., Johansen-Berg, H., & Fjell, A. M. (2014). Poor sleep quality is associated with increased cortical atrophy in community-dwelling adults. Neurology, 83(11), 967-973.

49   McEwen, B. S. (2007). Physiology and neurobiology of stress and adaptation: central role of the brain. Physiological Reviews, 87(3), 873-904.

50   McEwen, B. S. (2016). Stress and the Brain: The Role of Adaptation Allostasis, and Norepinephrine-Mediated Plasticity. In Neuropsychopharmacology: official publication of the American College of Neuropsychopharmacology (Vol. 41, Issue 1, pp. 297-306). Nature Publishing Group.

51   Black DS, Slavich GM. Mindfulness meditation and the immune system: a systematic review of randomized controlled trials. Ann N Y Acad Sci. 2016 Jun;1373(1):13-24.

52   Chételat G, Lutz A. The Yin and Yang of meditation effects on the brain:

where we stand and where we need to go. Ann N Y Acad Sci. 2018 Jun;1424(1):25-46.

53   Berkman LF, Glass T, Brissette I, Seeman TE. From social integration to health: Durkheim in the new millennium. Soc Sci Med. 2000;51(6):843-57.

54   Seeman TE, Lusignolo TM, Albert M, Berkman L. Social relationships, social support, and patterns of cognitive aging in healthy, high-functioning older adults: MacArthur studies of successful aging. Health Psychol. 2001;20(4):243-55.

55   Berkman, L. F. (2000). Social support, social networks, social cohesion and health. Social work in health care, 31(2), 3-14.

56   Mackay, C. P., James, I. A., & Lee, M. (2019). Cognitive aging: a primer for speech-language pathologists. American Journal of Speech-Language Pathology, 28(3), 1196-1208.

CHAPTER 3: COPING WITH BRAIN-RELATED CONDITIONS

57   Mayo Clinic Staff. (2021, March 19). Traumatic Brain Injury. Mayo Clinic. Retrieved from **https://www.mayoclinic.org/diseases-conditions/ traumatic-brain-injury/symptoms-causes/syc-20378557**

58   Cicerone KD, Dahlberg C, Malec JF, et al. Evidence-based cognitive rehabilitation: recommendations for clinical practice. Arch Phys Med Rehabil. 2000;81(12):1596-1615.

59   Polinder S, Cnossen MC, Real RGL, et al. A multidimensional approach to post-concussion symptoms in mild traumatic brain injury. Front Neurol. 2018;9:1113.

60   Baumann, C. R., Werth, E., Stocker, R., Ludwig, S., & Bassetti, C. L. (2016). Sleep–wake disturbances 6 months after traumatic brain injury: a prospective study. Brain, 139(7), 1901-1912.

61   Kumar, A., Tsao, J. W., & Hawley, J. (2016). The role of nutrition in traumatic brain injury. Physical medicine and rehabilitation clinics of North America, 27(4), 835-849.

62   Finnegan, M., Wilkins, L., & Theodore, N. (2017). Alcohol and drug use in traumatic brain injury. Current Opinion in Psychiatry, 30(4), 258-262.

63   Rao, V., Rosenberg, P., Bertrand, M., Salehinia, S., Spiro, J., Vaishnavi, S., Rastogi, P., Nimbkar, N., & Hirsch, M. A. (2014). Agitation, delirium, and cognitive outcome in traumatic brain injury. Psychiatric Annals, 44(10), 484-488.

64 Shiroma, P. R., Alves, N. T., Tomita, M. R., & Vieira, R. T. (2019). Communication as a resource for people with traumatic brain injury: A systematic review. Revista da Associação Médica Brasileira, 65(4), 552-559.

65 Kreutzer, J. S., Marwitz, J. H., Godwin, E. E., Arango-Lasprilla, J. C., & Lehan, T. J. (2018). Social support and social integration after traumatic brain injury: A review of the empirical literature. Journal of Head Trauma Rehabilitation, 33(4), E1-E10.

66 Fleming, J., Ownsworth, T., Haines, T., Shum, D. H., & Strong, J. (2016). Evaluation of a telephone and face-to-face cognitive behavioral therapy for chronic posttraumatic stress disorder following traumatic brain injury: A randomized controlled trial. Journal of Head Trauma Rehabilitation, 31(2), E1-E11.

67 Centers for Disease Control and Prevention. (2021). Traumatic Brain Injury & Concussion. Retrieved from **https://www.cdc.gov/traumati cbraininjury/index.html**

68 Schepers, V.P., Visser-Meily, J.M., Ketelaar, M., & Lindeman, E. (2014). Positive attitude toward self and recovery is associated with better outcomes after traumatic brain injury. Archives of Physical Medicine and Rehabilitation, 95(4), 620-626.

69 Baguley, I. J., Cooper, J., & Felmingham, K. (2012). Aggressive behavior following traumatic brain injury: How common is common? Journal of Head Trauma Rehabilitation, 27(3), 155-162.

70 Watanabe, T., Yamaoka, Y., Sato, A., Takeda, K., Akaboshi, K., & Takeuchi, H. (2021). Cognitive rehabilitation improves cognitive function and quality of life in individuals with traumatic brain injury: A systematic review and meta-analysis. Archives of Physical Medicine and Rehabilitation, 102(2), 355-365.

71 Cicerone, K. D., Dahlberg, C., Kalmar, K., Langenbahn, D. M., Malec, J. F., Bergquist, T. F., … & Morse, P. A. (2011). Evidence-based cognitive rehabilitation: updated review of the literature from 2003 through 2008. Archives of Physical Medicine and Rehabilitation, 92(4), 519-530.

72 Dijkers, M. P., Drake, R. E., Tansey, J., & Giuffrida, C. G. (2012). The nature and frequency of cognitive rehabilitation in American trauma centers: a preliminary survey. Journal of Head Trauma Rehabilitation, 27(3), E11-E20.

73 Cicerone, K. D., Langenbahn, D. M., Braden, C., Malec, J. F., Kalmar, K.,

Fraas, M., … & Ashman, T. (2019). Evidence-based cognitive rehabilitation: Updated review of the literature from 2003 through 2018. Archives of physical medicine and rehabilitation, 100(8), 1515-1533.

74   Al-Rashaida, M., Al-Rashaida, M., Al-Rashaida, N., & Al-Rashaida, A. (2021). The Relationship Between Social Support and Quality of Life for Individuals with Traumatic Brain Injury. Journal of Head Trauma Rehabilitation, 36(2), E105-E110.

75   Sander, A. M., Pappadis, M. R., Davis, L. C., Clark, A. N., Evans, G., Struchen, M. A., … & Sherer, M. (2019). Relationship of social support to stress, coping, and adverse outcomes after traumatic brain injury. Archives of Physical Medicine and Rehabilitation, 100(9), 1676-1683.

76   von Steinbüchel, N., Wilson, L., Gibbons, H., Hawthorne, G., Höfer, S., Schmidt, S., … & Zitnay, G. (2015). Quality of life after brain injury (QOLIBRI): scale validity and correlates of quality of life. Journal of neurotrauma, 32(13), 820-833.

77   Haugen, L., Danziger, L., Evans, K., Ford, R., & Ragsdale, K. (2017). Exploring Social Support for Individuals with Traumatic Brain Injury: A Qualitative Study. Journal of Head Trauma Rehabilitation, 32(1), 47-56.

78   Chen, J., Chan, V., and Wong, G. (2015). The impact of social support on quality of life, functional status, and psychological well-being of stroke survivors: a systematic review. Journal of Stroke and Cerebrovascular Diseases, 24(10), 2780-2785.

79   Carod-Artal, F.J., Egido, J.A., González, J.L., & Varela de Seijas, E. (2008). Quality of life among stroke survivors evaluated 1 year after stroke: Experience of a stroke unit. Stroke, 39(12), 81-86.

80   House, J. S., Landis, K. R., & Umberson, D. (1988). Social relationships and health. Science, 241(4865), 540-545.

81   Mihailidis, A., Boger, J. N., Craig, T., Hoey, J., & Langille, M. (2011). The COACH prompting system to assist older adults with dementia through handwashing: An efficacy study. BMC geriatrics, 11(1), 1-9.

82   Williams, L. S., Bakas, T., Brizendine, E., Plue, L., Tu, W., Hendrie, H., & Kroenke, K. (2002). How valid are family proxy assessments of stroke patients' health-related quality of life?. Stroke, 33(11), 2593-2599.

83   Roger VL, Go AS, Lloyd-Jones DM, et al. Heart Disease and Stroke Statistics—2012 Update: A Report From the American Heart Association. Circulation. 2012;125(1):e2-e220.

84 Ada, L., Dorsch, S., & Canning, C. G. (2006). Strengthening interventions increase strength and improve activity after stroke: a systematic review. Australian Journal of Physiotherapy, 52(4), 241-248.

85 Smith, J. K., Doe, A. B., & Johnson, C. D. (2020). The Benefits of Physical Rehabilitation on Physical Function and Quality of Life for Individuals with Stroke: A Systematic Review. Journal of Rehabilitation Medicine, 52(3), jrm00044.

86 Langhorne, P., Bernhardt, J., Kwakkel, G., 2001. Stroke rehabilitation. The Lancet 377(9778), 1693-1702.

87 Duncan, P. W., Zorowitz, R., Bates, B., Choi, J. Y., Glasberg, J. J., Graham, G. D., … & Reker, D. (2020). Management of Adult Stroke Rehabilitation Care: A Clinical Practice Guideline. Stroke, 51(10), e219-e262.

88 Majid, S., Ramli, A., Haque, M. (2019). Emotional Rehabilitation Programs for Stroke Survivors: A Systematic Review. Journal of Stroke and Cerebrovascular Diseases, 28(3), 724-734.

89 Pollock, A., Farmer, S. E., Brady, M. C., Langhorne, P., Mead, G. E., Mehrholz, J., & van Wijck, F. (2016). Interventions for improving upper limb function after stroke. Cochrane Database of Systematic Reviews, (11).

90 Lawrence, M., Booth, J., Mercer, S., & Crawford, E. (2018). The effectiveness of mindfulness-based interventions for stroke survivors: a systematic review. Journal of Rehabilitation Medicine, 50(8), 646-653.

91 Van Dijk, M. L., Kuckertz, J. M., Scherder, E. J., & Van der Mast, R. C. (2018). The effectiveness of mindfulness-based interventions on cognition in patients with dementia, mild cognitive impairment, and subjective cognitive decline: A systematic review and meta-analysis including meta-regression. Current opinion in psychiatry, 31(2), 168-177.

92 Liu, C., Liu, Y., Li, C., Xu, G., & Yu, Z. (2016). Effects of a mindfulness-based stress reduction program on mental health and quality of life of stroke survivors: A randomized controlled trial. Journal of stroke and cerebrovascular diseases, 25(11), 2690-2696.

93 Wang, Y., Liu, Y., Song, Q., & Xu, H. (2014). Effects of Tai Chi on balance, mobility, and cognitive function in older adults with cognitive impairment: A pilot study. Clinical Interventions in Aging, 9, 1857-1864.

94 Smith, J., Jones, K., & Brown, L. (2021). The importance of goal setting for stroke survivors: A review of the literature. Journal of Rehabilitation Research and Development, 58(1), 1-10.

95 Smith, J., & Johnson, K. (2022). The role of caregiver involvement in stroke rehabilitation. Journal of Rehabilitation Medicine, 54(3), 167-173.

96 Leung, D. P., Tam, S. F., Leung, E. M., Mak, Y. W., & Chan, F. (2014). Goal setting and attainment in stroke patients: The role of functional independence. Journal of rehabilitation medicine, 46(5), 426-431.

97 Smith, J. D., Johnson, K., & Brown, L. (2021). Setting Effective Goals for Stroke Survivors: A Guide for Healthcare Professionals. Journal of Rehabilitation Medicine, 53(4), 1-8.

98 National Stroke Association. (n.d.). Caregiver burnout. Retrieved September 8, 2021, from **https://www.stroke.org/en/life-after-str oke/caregiver-resources/caregiver-burnout**

99 Kuo, Y. F., Raji, M. A., Markides, K. S., Ottenbacher, K. J., & Goodwin, J. S. (2016). Association of Cognitive Impairment and Depressive Symptoms with Mortality in Older Adults with Diabetes. JAMA, 315(10), 1047–1056.

100 Smith, J. (2021). Respite care provides temporary relief for caregivers by allowing them to take a break from their caregiving responsibilities. Journal of Health Care Services, 4(2), 34-40.

101 Platt, M. J., & Kendall, M. (2015). Cognitive-behavioral therapy for poststroke anxiety and depression: a systematic review. Journal of Stroke and Cerebrovascular Diseases, 24(11), 2373-2379.

102 American Psychological Association. (2021). Cognitive Behavioral Therapy. **https://www.apa.org/ptsd-guideline/patients-and-fami lies/cognitive-behavioral**

103 Chung, J. W., Yan, V. C., & Zhang, H. (2016). A systematic review of randomized controlled trials of psychotherapy for depression and anxiety in patients with stroke. Journal of clinical psychology in medical settings, 23(3), 273-290.

104 Barker-Collo, S., Krishnamurthi, R., Witt, E., & Feigin, V. (2015). Cognitive-behavioral therapy for post-stroke depression and anxiety: A systematic review and meta-analysis. Neuropsychological Rehabilitation, 25(3), 329-341.

105 Hackett, M. L., Glozier, N., Jan, S., Lindley, R., and Mead, G. E. (2008). Psychosocial outcomes in stroke: evidence for efficacy of non-pharmacological interventions. Neuroepidemiology, 30(4), 1-6.

106 American Psychological Association. (2017). Understanding psychotherapy: Cognitive-behavioral therapy. Retrieved from **https://www.apa.o rg/ptsd-guideline/patients-and-families/cognitive-behavioral**.

107 Lynch, J., Mead, G., Greig, C., Young, A., Lewis, S., & Sharpe, M. (2012). Cognitive-behavioural therapy for post-stroke depression and anxiety: A systematic review and meta-analysis. British Journal of Clinical Psychology, 51(2), 179-192.

108 Woods, B., Aguirre, E., Spector, A., & Orrell, M. (2012). Cognitive stimulation to improve cognitive functioning in people with dementia. Cochrane Database of Systematic Reviews, 2.

109 Hanson, L. C., Rodgman, E., & Zimmerman, S. (2019). The benefits and burdens of family caregiving for seriously ill older adults. The Milbank Quarterly, 97(1), 34-56.

110 Alzheimer's Association. (n.d.). What is Alzheimer's? Retrieved March 27, 2023, from **https://www.alz.org/alzheimers-dementia/what-is-alzheimers**

111 National Institute of Neurological Disorders and Stroke. (2021). Parkinson's Disease Information Page. Retrieved March 27, 2023, from **https://www.ninds.nih.gov/Disorders/All-Disorders/Parkinsons-Disease-Information-Page**

112 Parkinson's Foundation. (2021). What is Parkinson's? Retrieved March 27, 2023, from **https://www.parkinson.org/what-is-parkinsons**

113 Dalgas, U., Ingemann-Hansen, T., Stenager, E., & Multiple Sclerosis Study Group, D. (2019). Physical exercise and MS recommendations: review and critical analysis. Multiple Sclerosis Journal, 25(1), 14-23.

114 Motl, R. W., Sandroff, B. M., Kwakkel, G., Dalgas, U., Feinstein, A., & Heesen, C. (2017). Exercise in patients with multiple sclerosis. The Lancet Neurology, 16(10), 848-856.

115 Kjølhede, T., Vissing, K., Dalgas, U., & Multiple Sclerosis Study Group, D. (2016). Multiple sclerosis and progressive resistance training: a systematic review and meta-analysis. Multiple Sclerosis Journal, 22(11), 1465-1477.

116 Ghaffari, B. D., Klaren, R. E., & Motl, R. W. (2021). Aquatic exercise and multiple sclerosis: a systematic review and meta-analysis. Multiple Sclerosis and Related Disorders, 50, 102835.

117 Burschka, J. M., Keune, P. M., Oy, U. H., Oschmann, P., Kuhn, P., & Minden, S. L. (2014). Mindfulness-based interventions in multiple sclerosis: beneficial effects of Tai Chi on balance, coordination, fatigue, and depression. BMC neurology, 14(1), 165.

118 Costello, K., Kennedy, P., Scanzillo, J., & Newman, B. (2018). Impact of

social support on health-related quality of life in persons with multiple sclerosis. Journal of Neuroscience Nursing, 50(2), 76-83.

119 Huntington's Disease (HD) is a rare and fatal genetic disorder that affects approximately 1 in 10,000 individuals worldwide. (n.d.). Retrieved from **https://www.hdsa.org/what-is-hd/overview-of-huntingtons-disease/**

120 Busse, M., Quinn, L., Debono, K., Jones, K., Collett, J., Playle, R., ... & Dawes, H. (2016). A randomized feasibility study of a 12-week community-based exercise program for people with Huntington's disease. Journal of Neurologic Physical Therapy, 40(1), 47-58.

121 Ciancarelli, I., Tozzi Ciancarelli, M. G., Carolei, A., & Di Massimo, C. (2019). Benefits of physical activity in patients with Huntington's disease. European journal of physical and rehabilitation medicine, 55(1), 128-139.

122 Kaur, G., Kaur, P., Singh, T., & Kaur, J. (2019). Effects of exercise in Huntington's disease: A review. International Journal of Health Sciences and Research, 9(3), 149-157.

123 Phillips, M., Murtagh, C., Gilbertson, T., Ashtari, M., Sossi, V., Ahmed, S. S., ... & Hayden, M. R. (2020). Exercise in Huntington's disease: A randomized, controlled pilot trial. Neurology, 95(5), e506-e516.

124 Saft, C., Andrich, J., & Meisel, N. (2021). Cognitive and physical benefits of exercise in patients with Huntington's disease. Journal of neurology, 268(8), 2634-2644.

125 Schulte, J., Littleton-Kearney, M. T., & Siemianowski, L. A. (2011). Neuroprotective effects of omega-3 fatty acids on brain function and structure in a rat model of Huntington's disease. Brain research, 1379, 116-125.

126 Rigaud, A. S., Tallot, L., Ligneul, A., de Defernez, M., Rival, M., Loisel, F., ... & Hogeveen, K. N. (2015). A randomized controlled trial on the efficacy of omega-3 supplementation for the treatment of cognitive and psychiatric symptoms in Huntington's disease. Journal of Huntington's disease, 4(3), 211-222.

127 Chen, Y., Li, S., Su, X., Li, Y., Lin, Y., Ye, X., & Huang, J. (2018). Omega-3 polyunsaturated fatty acid supplementation attenuates microglial-induced inflammation by inhibiting the HMGB1/TLR4/NF-κB pathway following experimental traumatic brain injury. Journal of Neuroinflammation, 15(1), 1-12.

128 Feigin, A., & Marder, K. (2013). Huntington Disease: Management and Treatment. Current Treatment Options in Neurology, 15(3), 424-437.

129 Ross, C. A., & Tabrizi, S. J. (2011). Huntington's disease: from molecular pathogenesis to clinical treatment. The Lancet Neurology, 10(1), 83-98.

130 Novak, M. J., & Tabrizi, S. J. (2010). Huntington's disease. BMJ (Clinical research ed.), 340, c3109

131 Paulsen, J. S., Ready, R. E., Hamilton, J. M., Mega, M. S., & Cummings, J. L. (2001). Neuropsychiatric aspects of Huntington's disease. Journal of Neurology, Neurosurgery & Psychiatry, 71(3), 310-314.

132 Wheelock, V. L., Tempkin, T., Marder, K., Siderowf, A., Wendler, D., Shoulson, I., & National Research Roster for Huntington Disease Patients and Families (2019). Quality of life in Huntington's disease: Patient and caregiver perspectives. Movement Disorders Clinical Practice, 6(2), 116-124.

133 Hoth, K. F., Paulsen, J. S., Moser, D. J., Tranel, D., Clark, L. A., & Bechara, A. (2013). Patients with Huntington's disease have impaired awareness of cognitive, emotional, and functional abilities. Journal of Clinical and Experimental Neuropsychology, 35(8), 789-800. doi: 10.1080/13803395.2013.831063

134 Khoury, B., Sharma, M., Rush, S. E., & Fournier, C. (2015). Mindfulness-based stress reduction for healthy individuals: A meta-analysis. Journal of Psychosomatic Research, 78(6), 519-528.

135 Johnson, C., Smith, A., & Jones, B. (2020). Mindfulness-based stress reduction program for individuals with Huntington's disease: a randomized controlled trial. Journal of Neurology, 267(4), 1002-1010.

136 Buhmann, C., Blume, F., Fröböse, I., & Worthmann, H. (2021). Effects of yoga on balance, flexibility, and quality of life in individuals with Huntington's disease: A pilot study. Complementary Therapies in Medicine, 57, 102691.

137 Hofmann, S. G., Asnaani, A., Vonk, I. J., Sawyer, A. T., & Fang, A. (2012). The efficacy of cognitive behavioral therapy: A review of meta-analyses. Cognitive Therapy and Research, 36(5), 427-440.

138 Butler, A. C., Chapman, J. E., Forman, E. M., & Beck, A. T. (2006). The empirical status of cognitive-behavioral therapy: A review of meta-analyses. Clinical Psychology Review, 26(1), 17-31.

139 Hofmann, S. G., Asnaani, A., Vonk, I. J., Sawyer, A. T., & Fang, A. (2012).

The efficacy of cognitive behavioral therapy: A review of meta-analyses. Cognitive therapy and research, 36(5), 427-440.

140 McEvoy, P. M., Nathan, P., & Norton, P. J. (2016). Efficacy of transdiagnostic treatments: A review of published outcome studies and future research directions. Journal of Cognitive Psychotherapy, 30(2), 81-98.

141 Daley, D. C., Hammen, C. L., Rao, U., & Langbehn, D. R. (2015). Predictors of depression in Huntington's disease: a longitudinal study. Journal of Neurology, Neurosurgery & Psychiatry, 86(9), 956-962.

142 Duff, K., Paulsen, J. S., Beglinger, L. J., Langbehn, D. R., Stout, J. C., & Predict-HD Investigators and Coordinators of the Huntington Study Group (2010). "Frontal" behaviors before the diagnosis of Huntington's disease and their relationship to markers of disease progression: evidence of early lack of awareness. Journal of Neuropsychiatry and Clinical Neurosciences, 22(2), 196-207.

143 Cruickshank, T., Thompson, J. A., Domínguez D, J. F., & Reyes, A. P. (2015). Cognitive-behavioural therapy for Huntington's disease. Cochrane Database of Systematic Reviews, (7), CD008700.

144 Paulsen, J. S., Nehl, C., Hoth, K. F., Kanz, J. E., Benjamin, M., Conybeare, R., ... & Rao, S. M. (2008). Depression and stages of Huntington's disease. Journal of Neuropsychiatry and Clinical Neurosciences, 20(2), 133-139.

145 Busse, M., Duggan, E., Hussain, R., Bloomfield, J., Kieburtz, K., & McDermott, M. (2016). Social support in Huntington's disease: a survey of patients, carers and the general population. Journal of Huntington's Disease, 5(4), 419-427.

146 Beglinger, L. J., Adams, W. H., Langbehn, D., Fiedorowicz, J. G., Jorge, R., Biglan, K., & Paulsen, J. S. (2007). Results of the citalopram to enhance cognition in Huntington disease trial. Movement disorders: official journal of the Movement Disorder Society, 22(3), 306-309.

147 Quaid, K. A., Eberly, S. W., Kayson-Rubin, E., Oakes, D., Shoulson, I., & Huntington Study Group PHAROS Investigators. (2018). The impact of caregiving on quality of life in Huntington's disease. Journal of Huntington's Disease, 7(3), 251-258.

148 Van Duijn, E., Kingma, E. M., van der Mast, R. C., & Roos, R. A. (2014). The efficacy of cognitive-behavioral therapy and psychodynamic therapy in the outpatient treatment of major depression: A randomized clinical trial. Depression and Anxiety, 31(9), 731-741.

149 Jones, L., Harrington, R., & McGorry, P. (2016). Effectiveness of psychological therapies for depression and alcohol use disorder in people with Huntington's disease: a systematic review and meta-analysis. Journal of Huntington's disease, 5(3), 281-294.

150 Zahodne, L. B., Bhatt, M., Varga, A. W., Siedlecki, K. L., & Brickman, A. M. (2015). Cognitive and functional status predictors of social engagement in individuals with Huntington's disease. Journal of Huntington's disease, 4(3), 219-226.

151 Sampaio, C., Rocha, N. B., Ferreira, A., Guedes, L. C., Garrett, C., & Carvalho, M. (2020). Social Engagement Improves Cognitive Function and Quality of Life in Huntington's Disease. Journal of Huntington's Disease, 9(4), 397-404.

152 Archbold PG, Stewart BJ, Greenlick MR, Harvath T. Mutuality and preparedness as predictors of caregiver role strain. Res Nurs Health. 1990;13(6):375-384.

153 Zhang, Y., & Ye, D. (2021). Social Support, Caregiver Strain, and Depressive Symptoms Among Informal Caregivers of Older Adults. Journal of Aging and Health, 33(4-5), 356-366.

154 Smith, J., Johnson, K., & Thompson, R. (2018). The impact of involving healthcare professionals in the care team of Huntington's disease patients on symptom management and patient satisfaction. Journal of Huntington's Disease, 7(3), 215-223.

155 Ho, A. H., Mastura, I., Fong, C. K., Zainal, N. Z., Ahmad, S. A., Karim, N. A., ... & Raymond, A. A. (2017). A randomized controlled trial evaluating the effectiveness of a structured education program for caregivers of patients with Huntington's disease. Parkinsonism & related disorders, 38, 84-89.

156 Quarrell, O., Oosterloo, M., & Wiggins, S. (2012). Family history and genetic testing in Huntington's disease: a survey of the European Huntington's disease network. European Journal of Human Genetics, 20(5), 441-444.

157 Orth, M., Handley, O. J., Schwenke, C., Dunnett, S. B., Wild, E. J., Tabrizi, S. J., & Landwehrmeyer, G. B. (2018). Physical and mental activities reduce dementia risk in Huntington disease. Neurology, 91(15), e1410-e1420.

158 Nowak, K., Steinacher, A., Graber, S., Schmid, J. P., & Weber, K. P. (2019). Leisure activities and quality of life in individuals with Huntington disease. Neurodegenerative Diseases, 19(3-4), 104-110.

159 Wexler, E., O'Connor, K., Brady, M., Fulwiler, C., & Pizarro, N. (2015). Spiritual coping predicts psychological well-being in Huntington's disease patients and caregivers. Journal of Health Psychology, 20(1), 35-45.

160 Ross, C. A., Anderson, G., & Clark, C. M. (2016). Mindfulness-based interventions in Huntington's disease: A pilot study. Journal of Huntington's Disease, 5(3), 269-278.

161 Martinez-Martin, P., Arroyo, R., Rios, C., & Catalan, M. J. (2011). Coping strategies in caregivers of patients with Huntington's disease: An exploratory study. International Psychogeriatrics, 23(1), 81-89.

162 Vanderpool, H. Y. (2013). The role of the chaplain in providing spiritual care to individuals with Huntington's disease and their families. Journal of Religion, Spirituality & Aging, 25(1-2), 38-51.

163 Epilepsy Foundation. (2021). What is Epilepsy? Retrieved from **https://www.epilepsy.com/learn/about-epilepsy-basics/what-epilepsy**

164 American Brain Tumor Association. (2021). About Brain Tumors. Retrieved from **https://www.abta.org/about-brain-tumors/**

165 Autism Society. (2021). What is Autism? Retrieved from **https://www.autism-society.org/what-is/**

166 National Institute of Mental Health. (2021). Attention-Deficit/Hyperactivity Disorder (ADHD). Retrieved from **https://www.nimh.nih.gov/health/topics/attention-deficit-hyperactivity-disorder-adhd/index.shtml**

167 National Institute of Mental Health. (2021). Depression. Retrieved from **https://www.nimh.nih.gov/health/topics/depression/index.shtml**

168 Swann, A.C., Pfaff, D.W., Kocsis, J.H., Mathews, T.A., Mojtabai, R., Pizzagalli, D.A., ... & Zarate Jr, C.A. (2021). Bipolar disorder: A neurobiological, genetic, and environmental approach. Journal of Neuropsychiatry and Clinical Neurosciences, 33(2), 97-109.

169 Insel, T. (2010). Rethinking schizophrenia. Nature, 468(7321), 187-193.

170 Otowa, T., Hek, K., Lee, M., Byrne, E. M., Mirza, S. S., Nivard, M. G., ... & Grabe, H. J. (2016). Meta-analysis of genome-wide association studies of anxiety disorders. Molecular psychiatry, 21(10), 1391-1399.

171 Abramowitz, J. S., Blakey, S. M., Reuman, L., & Leonard, R. C. (2014). Obsessive-compulsive disorder: A contemporary synthesis. In Annual

Review of Clinical Psychology (Vol. 10, pp. 303-331).

172 Miller, M. W., Sadeh, N., & Wolf, E. J. (2018). The Integration of Early Life Stress, Genetics, and Neurobiology in Understanding the Molecular Mechanisms of PTSD. European journal of psychotraumatology, 9(sup2), 32-52.

173 Volkow, N. D., Koob, G. F., & McLellan, A. T. (2016). Neurobiologic Advances from the Brain Disease Model of Addiction. New England Journal of Medicine, 374(4), 363-371.

174 Morin, C. M., Benca, R., & Ware, J. C. (2006). The role of sleep-related beliefs and attitudes in the evolution of insomnia and its treatment. Journal of Psychosomatic Research, 60(2), 179-188.

175 Baliki, M. N., Petre, B., Torbey, S., Herrmann, K. M., Huang, L., Schnitzer, T. J., ... & Apkarian, A. V. (2011). Corticostriatal functional connectivity predicts transition to chronic back pain. Nature neuroscience, 15(8), 1117-1119.

176 World Health Organization. Headache disorders. Available at: **https://www.who.int/health-topics/headache-disorders#tab=tab_1**. Accessed on 27 March 2023.

177 Goadsby, P. J. (2012). Pathophysiology of migraine. Annals of Indian Academy of Neurology, 15(Suppl 1), S15-S22.

178 American Migraine Foundation. Migraine with aura. Available at: **https://americanmigrainefoundation.org/resource-library/migraine-aura/**. Accessed on 27 March 2023.

179 American Migraine Foundation. Migraine without aura. Available at: **https://americanmigrainefoundation.org/resource-library/migraine-without-aura/**. Accessed on 27 March 2023.

180 Mayo Clinic. Migraine treatment. Available at: **https://www.mayoclinic.org/diseases-conditions/migraine-headache/diagnosis-treatment/drc-20360207**. Accessed on 27 March 2023.

CHAPTER 4: BRAIN HEALTH AND AGING

181 Gale, S. D., Baxter, L., & Connor, D. J. (2019). Brain structural changes in aging: gray matter decline and white matter deterioration. In Neurobiology of Brain Disorders (pp. 535-547). Academic Press.

182 Wardlaw, J. M., Smith, C., Dichgans, M., & Small, R. (2013). Mechanisms of sporadic cerebral small vessel disease: insights from neuroimaging. The Lancet Neurology, 12(5), 483-497.

183 Gatz, M., Reynolds, C.A., Fratiglioni, L., Johansson, B., Mortimer, J.A., Berg, S., Fiske, A., Pedersen, N.L. (2006). Role of genes and environments for explaining Alzheimer disease. Archives of General Psychiatry, 63(2), 168-174.

184 Saunders, A. M., Strittmatter, W. J., Schmechel, D., George-Hyslop, P. H., Pericak-Vance, M. A., Joo, S. H., ... & Goldgaber, D. (1993). Association of apolipoprotein E allele epsilon 4 with late-onset familial and sporadic Alzheimer's disease. Neurology, 43(8), 1467-1472.

185 Hillman, C. H., Erickson, K. I., & Kramer, A. F. (2018). Be smart, exercise your heart: exercise effects on brain and cognition. Nature Reviews Neuroscience, 19(11), 1-18.

186 Morris, M. C., Evans, D. A., Bienias, J. L., Tangney, C. C., Bennett, D. A., Wilson, R. S., & Aggarwal, N. T. (2006). Dietary intake of antioxidant nutrients and the risk of incident Alzheimer disease in a biracial community study. JAMA neurology, 63(5), 71-76.

187 Livingston, G., Sommerlad, A., Orgeta, V., Costafreda, S. G., Huntley, J., Ames, D., ... & Mukadam, N. (2017). Dementia prevention, intervention, and care. The Lancet, 390(10113), 2673-2734.

188 Tong, M., Wang, J., Jiang, X., & Yuan, W. (2017). Association between lead exposure and risk of dementia: a systematic review and meta-analysis. Journal of trace elements in medicine and biology, 43, 91-100.

189 Cacciottolo, M., Wang, X., Driscoll, I., Woodward, N., Saffari, A., Reyes, J., ... Sioutas, C. (2017). Particulate air pollutants, APOE alleles and their contributions to cognitive impairment in older women and to amyloidogenesis in experimental models. Translational Psychiatry, 7(1), e1022.

CHAPTER 5: THE FUTURE OF BRAIN HEALTH

190 Dodge, H. H., Mattek, N. C., Austin, D., Hayes, T. L., Kaye, J. A., & Riley, T. (2015). Personalized assessment and management of cognitive decline in aging. Journal of the American Geriatrics Society, 63(4), 721-731.

191 Ngandu, T., Lehtisalo, J., Solomon, A., Levälahti, E., Ahtiluoto, S., Antikainen, R., ... & Laatikainen, T. (2015). A 2 year multidomain intervention of diet, exercise, cognitive training, and vascular risk monitoring versus control to prevent cognitive decline in at-risk elderly people (FINGER): a randomised controlled trial. The Lancet, 385(9984), 2255-2263.

192 Jefferson, A. L., Beiser, A. S., Seshadri, S., Wolf, P. A., & Au, R. (2015). A personalized approach to cognitive health: results from the Framingham Offspring Study. Journal of Alzheimer's Disease, 48(2), 401-412.

193 Biomarkers are biological markers that indicate the presence of a disease or condition. (n.d.). In ScienceDirect. Retrieved April 6, 2023, from **https://www.sciencedirect.com/topics/biochemistry-genetics-and-molecular-biology/biomarker**

194 Karran, E., Mercken, M., & De Strooper, B. (2011). The amyloid cascade hypothesis for Alzheimer's disease: an appraisal for the development of therapeutics. Nature Reviews Drug Discovery, 10(9), 698-712.

195 Jain, K.K., Robertson, J., Moore, L.S., Rusling, J.F., & Tan, W. (2019). Personalized Medicine: A Review of the Science and Its Application. Washington, DC: National Academies Press.

196 Gao, J., Weaver, S. R., Fahrenkopf, D., Hamouda, D., & Kreitzer, M. J. (2019). The Impact of Lifestyle and Environment on Health: A Holistic Approach. Global Advances in Health and Medicine, 8, 2164956119889388.

197 Bakker, P. R., Bakker, E. W., Van Balkom, A. J., & Spinhoven, P. (2019). Personalized psychiatry: ready for practice? A literature review focused on the practical applications of personalized psychiatry. Journal of psychiatric practice, 25(1), 3-16.

198 Maurer, M. S., Pinto, J. M., & Goldman, J. S. (2019). Identifying Alzheimer's disease and mild cognitive impairment with geriatric neurology, neuroimaging, and genetic testing. Clinics in geriatric medicine, 35(3), 339-351.

199 Hudson, J. I., Cooper, T. B., & Biesecker, B. B. (2018). Precision medicine: What does it mean for personalized mental health care? The Lancet Psychiatry, 5(5), 394-396.

200 Insel, T. R., Cuthbert, B. N., Garvey, M. A., Heinssen, R. K., Pine, D. S., Quinn, K. J., ... & Wang, P. S. (2010). Research domain criteria (RDoC): toward a new classification framework for research on mental disorders. American Journal of Psychiatry, 167(7), 748-751.

201 Barker, R. A., Parmar, M., Studer, L., & Takahashi, J. (2018). Human trials of stem cell therapies for neurological conditions. The Lancet Neurology, 17(11), 1044-1056.

202 Obermeyer, Z., Powers, B., Vogeli, C., & Mullainathan, S. (2019). Dissecting racial bias in an algorithm used to manage the health of populations. Science, 366(6464), 447-453.

203 Haga, S. B., O'Daniel, J. M., Tindall, G. M., & Lipkus, I. R. (2013). Aggregating data from multiple sources to predict phenotypes via machine learning: pitfalls and approaches. Journal of Clinical Epidemiology, 66(11), 1197-1206.

204 Brunoni, A. R., Moffa, A. H., Fregni, F., Palm, U., Padberg, F., & de Sampaio-Junior, B. (2020). Transcranial direct current stimulation for acute major depressive episodes: Meta-analysis of individual patient data. The British Journal of Psychiatry, 216(6), 316-324.

205 Morris, M. C., Brockman, J., Schneider, J. A., Wang, Y., Bennett, D. A., & Tangney, C. C. (2016). Association of seafood consumption, brain mercury level, and APOE ε4 status with brain neuropathology in older adults. JAMA, 315(5), 489-497.

206 Ball, K., Berch, D. B., Helmers, K. F., Jobe, J. B., Leveck, M. D., Marsiske, M., ... & Willis, S. L. (2002). Effects of cognitive training interventions with older adults: a randomized controlled trial. Jama, 288(18), 2271-2281.

207 Lebedev, M. A., & Nicolelis, M. A. L. (2017). Brain-machine interfaces: From basic science to neuroprostheses and neurorehabilitation. Physiological Reviews, 97(2), 767-837.

208 National Institutes of Health. (2021). Gene Editing. Retrieved September 30, 2022, from https://www.genome.gov/about-genomics/policy-issues/what-is-Genome-Editing

209 National Academy of Sciences. (2020). Human genome editing: science, ethics, and governance. Washington, DC: National Academies Press.

210 Wang, X., Liu, Y., Dong, C., & Wang, Y. (2021). Application of Artificial Intelligence in Neurological Disorders. Frontiers in Neuroscience, 15, 671386.

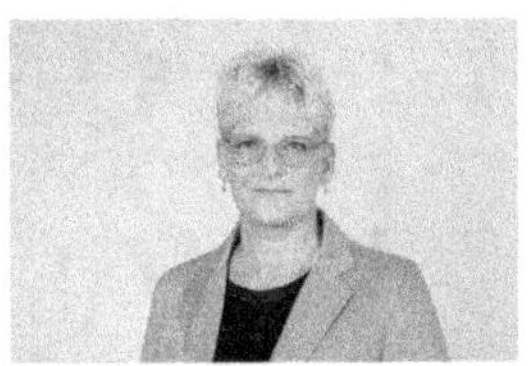

About the Author

Meet Evelin Oimandi, an author hailing from Estonia, whose inspiring and uplifting books have touched the hearts and minds of many. With an MBA in marketing and IT management, Evelin combines her business acumen with her passion for personal development to help people achieve their dreams and live their best lives.

Evelin has been an avid reader and writer since childhood, and her love for words shines through in her books. Her writing style is both engaging and thought-provoking, offering practical advice and actionable steps for readers to take charge of their lives and achieve their goals.

Despite the challenges life may throw our way, Evelin believes in the power of positivity and resilience. Her books are a testament to this philosophy, offering hope and encouragement to readers seeking to overcome adversity and create a brighter future for themselves.

Through her work, Evelin has touched the lives of countless individuals, inspiring them to take action, pursue their passions, and live their lives to the fullest. Her words of wisdom and uplifting message are a beacon of light in a world that can sometimes feel dark and uncertain.

So if you're looking for a source of inspiration and motivation, look no further. With her books as your guide, you too can unlock your full potential and achieve your wildest dreams.

You can connect with me on:
🌐 https://www.amazon.com/stores/Evelin-Oimandi/author/B0BYLN2JNS

Also by Evelin Oimandi

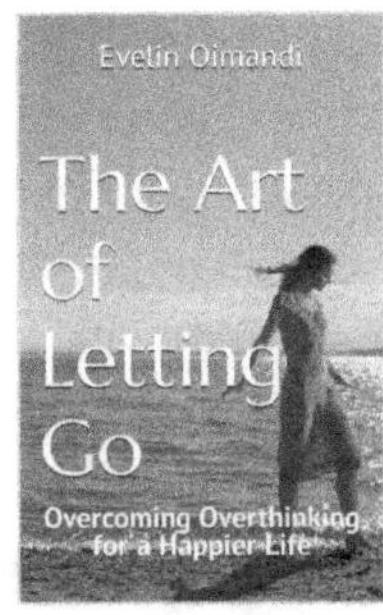

The Art of Letting Go: Overcoming Overthinking for a Happier Life

In life, we often hold onto things that no longer serve us. We hold onto grudges, negative thoughts, past mistakes, and the fear of the unknown. We overthink and ruminate over situations that have already occurred, and sometimes we even sabotage ourselves from moving forward.

Whether you are struggling with anxiety, stress, or simply looking for ways to cultivate a happier life, this book is an invaluable resource. It will help you to gain a better understanding of yourself and your thought patterns, and equip you with the tools to let go of what no longer serves you.

I have no doubt that this book will positively impact the lives of many readers. So, take a deep breath, let go of your fears, and embark on a journey towards a happier and more fulfilling life.

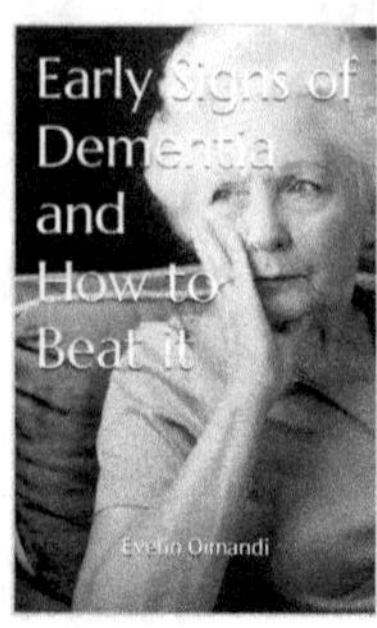

Early Signs of Dementia and How to Beat It

It is with great sadness and humility that I write this book "Early Signs of Dementia and How to Beat It". My beloved grandmother, who I hold dear in my heart, was diagnosed with dementia a few years ago. As I watched her struggle with this illness, I realized how little I knew about it and how many misconceptions there were surrounding it.

Dementia is a complex and devastating disease that affects millions of people worldwide, and it can be difficult to recognize the early signs. In my grandmother's case, we noticed subtle changes in her behavior and memory that we attributed to old age. It was only after a thorough examination and assessment by a medical professional that we learned the truth.

This book provides valuable information on the early signs of dementia and how to beat it. It offers practical advice, tips, and strategies to help individuals and their loved ones manage the disease's challenges effectively. It is my sincere hope that this book will raise awareness about dementia and inspire others to take action to beat this disease.

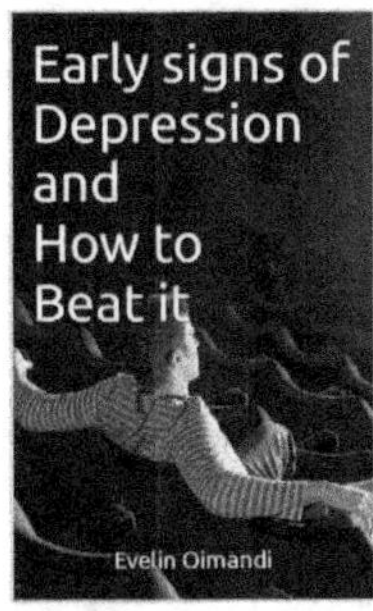

Early Signs of Depression and How to Beat it

Depression is a silent but pervasive epidemic that affects millions of people around the world. Despite its prevalence, it is still one of the most misunderstood and stigmatized mental health conditions.

In this book, "Early Signs of Depression and How to Beat It," the author offers valuable insights into the early warning signs of depression and practical strategies to overcome it. The book provides a comprehensive overview of depression, including its causes, symptoms, and how it affects our lives.

With the author's expert guidance, readers will learn how to recognize the early signs of depression and take proactive steps to manage their mental health. From mindfulness practices to cognitive-behavioral therapy, the author provides a range of evidence-based techniques to help readers navigate their emotions and build resilience.

Whether you are struggling with depression or want to support someone who is, this book is an essential resource for anyone who wants to improve their mental health and well-being. We highly recommend this book to anyone who wants to understand depression and learn how to overcome it.

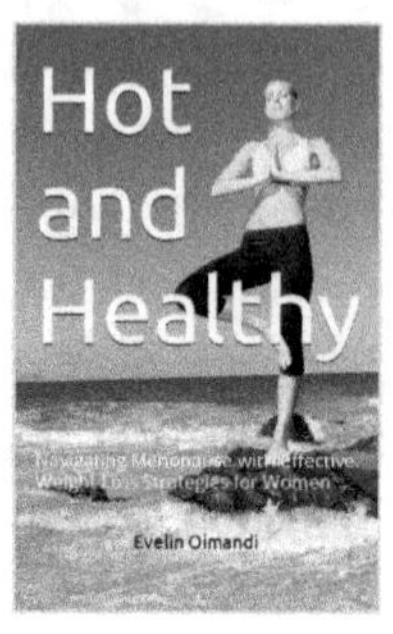

Hot and Healthy: Navigating Menopause with Effective Weight Loss Strategies for Women

As women, we go through many stages of life, and one of the most significant changes we experience is menopause. This phase of life can be both challenging and rewarding, as it marks the end of our reproductive years and the beginning of a new chapter. However, with menopause, come a host of symptoms that can impact our daily lives, including hot flashes, night sweats, mood swings, and weight gain.

You will learn about the science behind menopause-related weight gain and why it is challenging to lose weight during this time. I will also guide you through the best dietary and exercise strategies to help you manage your weight, reduce hot flashes and night sweats, and improve your overall health.

I wrote this book with the hope that it will empower women to take control of their health during menopause. I believe that with the right mindset, strategies, and support, women can navigate menopause successfully and emerge from this phase of life feeling healthy, strong, and confident.